Minding the Body
Clinical Uses
of Somatic Awareness

Donald Bakal

THE GUILFORD PRESS
New York   London

©1999 The Guilford Press
A Division of Guilford Publications, Inc.
72 Spring Street, New York, NY 10012
http://www.guilford.com

Printed in the United States of America

This book is printed on acid-free paper.

Last digit is print number: 9 8 7 6 5 4 3 2

Library of Congress Cataloging-in-Publication Data

Bakal, Donald
   Minding the body: clinical uses of somatic awareness /
Donald Bakal.
      p. cm.
   Includes bibliographical references and index.
   ISBN 1-57230-435-9 (hc.) 1-67230-661-0 (pbk.)
   1. Medicine, Psychosomatic. 2. Mind and Body. 3. Holistic
medicine.   I. Title.
   [DNLM: 1. Holistic Health. 2. Mind–Body Relations
(Metaphysics) 3. Alternative Medicine.   W 61 B166m
1999]
RC49.B34 1999
616′.001′9–dc21
DNLM/DLC
for Library of Congress   98-55170
                                                                      CIP

MINDING THE BODY

About the Author

Donald Bakal, PhD, is a professor of psychology at the University of Calgary in Alberta, Canada, and a geriatric clinical consultant with the Calgary Regional Health Authority. Widely published in the fields of behavioral medicine and health psychology, he is well known for his psychobiological model of chronic headache disorders.

Contents

MINDING THE BODY

CHAPTER 1

The Nature of Somatic Awareness

HOLISTIC HEALTH THROUGH BODY EXPERIENCE

Over the span of a few decades, health care has evolved from a singular faith in biomedicine and technology to recognition of the biopsychosocial nature of all illness. The shift from the biomedical to the biopsychosocial paradigm in medicine has been characterized, at both the scientific and the clinical levels, by far greater appreciation of *humanness* (Engel, 1997). "Humanness" refers in large part to the fact that we are capable of examining and regulating our own inner life and experience. There is considerable evidence that individuals who are actively engaged in some form of self-regulation have an improved quality of life. These individuals take much greater responsibility for their health and also play a more active role in the decision-making process with their health care providers.

The quality of humanness derives from our ability to use words to express what we are observing in the outer world as well as what we are experiencing in our inner world. The fact that humans can look inward may seem obvious; after all, we are all aware of experiencing inner feelings and sensations. However, the fact that humans have the ability to identify a special set of inner bodily experiences that can be used to prevent and manage illness is not obvious. This book provides a unique framework to help individuals understand what they can do within themselves to maintain health and to maximize their chances of recovery should they become ill. It is my thesis that such an internal state exists and that this state, which I call "somatic awareness," can be readily activated by all individuals on their own terms and circumstance to facilitate health.

Most health professionals, whether explicitly "holistic" or not, acknowledge that the biopsychosocial perspective contributes to a better understanding of their patients' problems. They recognize at an intellectual level that most of their patients' presenting symptoms have biological, psychological, and social aspects. The Center for Advancement of Health in Washington, DC (http://www.cfah.org), for example, has made the following recommendations for the holistic changes needed in health care:

1. Medical intervention must include recognition of how intimately health is linked to attitudes, thoughts, feelings, and behaviors.
2. Scientific evidence cannot be ignored—who we are, where we live, and how we think, feel, and cope with bodily information can powerfully influence whether we get sick, how sick we get, and how best to manage our illness.
3. Holistic patient management requires that patients not be sent to one "repair shop" for sick thoughts and feelings and to another "repair shop" for diseased organs. The mind and body flourish or perish together.
4. Patient care must shift to treating the whole person—the payoff will be healthier individuals, healthier communities, and a healthier nation. To do otherwise is irresponsible.

The problem facing health professionals, especially physicians, is how to achieve these objectives in clinical practice. Most physicians would welcome some guidance in using this model within the constraints of their daily medical practice. Most would agree that it would be more rewarding to share a patient's bodily experiences with an illness than to attempt to reduce the illness to objective biological observations alone. However, they still find it necessary to keep the biological and the psychosocial aspects of their patients' illnesses separate. That is, they problem-solve in one domain only and "graft on" the other domain as needed. Traditionally, physicians have been trained to isolate physical symptoms from psychosocial inputs. The patient's "physical" problems are dealt with within a biomedical framework, while the "patient" is referred to a psychologist for psychological problems, to a marital therapist for marital problems, and so on.

But successfully employing an integrated approach with patients means more than simply attending to their psychosocial concerns in addition to their medical concerns. Foss (1996) believes that today we are at a fork in the road in health care, with the biomedical and the biopsychosocial paradigms producing quite different and antithetical views of how best to treat patients:

> One choice is the choice of biomedicine, which holds that the patient is a biological organism, a mindless lifebody, such that the patient's psychology has no medically significant impact on physiology and disease is a deviation from the norm of somatic variables. . . . In the second alternative choice, the patient is an "articulate" mindbody, and disease is a deviation from the norm of psychosomatic or psychosociosomatic variables, over some of which the patient has limited control. . . . Logically there is no middle ground. Either the patient is only a biological, mindless entity or the patient is a "thinking" mindbody. One or the other. (p. 46)

There may be no middle ground between these views, but the biopsychosocial paradigm requires medical and psychosocial integration in practice. The psychobiological perspective must be practiced within reach of biomedicine. In cases of abdominal pain, unexplained headache, or other painful symptoms, the immediate origins of the pain can well be organic (e.g., infection, tumor). Regardless of whether an organic factor is identified, however, all health professionals involved in treating the patient need a perspective for understanding the patient's subjective and bodily experiences with the symptom. The pain may be partly or purely anxiety based—reflecting, for example, marital discord or fear of disease—or it may be driven by drug withdrawal or some other combination of factors. In the case of chronic illness, the issue becomes one of management rather than one of cure. Thus, it is critical that both health professionals and patients be willing to seek out bodily experiences that can be used to manage the accompanying symptoms.

It is no simple matter to link an approach that uses the "mind," that is, one based on our cognitive abilities, emotional responses, and the attitudes with which we meet experience, with an approach that uses biological and chemical entities that one way or another are made to enter the body (Dienstfrey, 1997). The largest unexplored problem in mind–body medicine is how to integrate its emerging treatments with the treatments of biochemical medicine. An experiential construct is needed to guide professionals and patients in their collaborative efforts to develop an integrated approach to psychobiological health.

I have worked as a behavioral scientist and a practitioner in the field of health psychology for more than 2 decades. Throughout this period I have followed a *psychobiological* approach that emphasizes the individual and the indivisible union of our physical and psychological realities (Bakal, 1992). I use the term "psychobiological" to reflect a holistic paradigm of the union of the psychological and the physiological processes involved in illness and health. My focus of study and of treatment has been the processes that mediate between psychological and physiological variables within the person rather than the processes that mediate between the person and his or her environment. In this book, I examine an experiential component of psychobiological health that I call somatic awareness. Somatic awareness is a difficult concept to describe. It is much easier to write about biopsychosocial and psychobiological issues than it is to capture inner experiences that reflect health and illness. But, although it is difficult to describe, the concept should be familiar to everyone.

Somatic awareness is at the cutting edge of the mind–body interface and represents a way to truly empower individuals in their efforts to maintain or restore good health. Somatic awareness constitutes an innate wisdom that people have about their own psychobiological health. It involves utilizing sensory information that is readily available, and that when utilized can contribute to all aspects of health, from preventing migraine, hypertension, and heart disease to regulating autoimmune diseases, and possibly to altering the course of cancer. For virtually all symptoms, diseases, and illness conditions, the mind's awareness of the body's sensations has a very significant role to play.

Somatic awareness is a commonplace inner experience. It is readily discernible in the background of consciousness. Although seldom made explicit in discussions of holistic health, its presence is implicit in virtually all forms of self-regulatory therapies, including relaxation, biofeedback, meditation, tai chi, and others. One definition of somatic awareness emphasizes the mental processes by which we perceive, interpret, and act on information from our bodies (Cioffi, 1991). Perception and interpretation *are* important aspects of bodily awareness but by themselves they do not necessarily lead to an integration of bodily information within consciousness. When somatic awareness is added to this view, however, inner awareness can be used to alleviate and prevent symptoms and to manage illness.

The familiar example of migraine headache can be used to illustrate the limitations of interpretation of painful symptoms is in isolation from integration. Suppose a person awakens with a headache. How he/she perceives or interprets this pain is critical to the course of this episode as well as to the course of future episodes. If the individual decides that the symptom is indicative of some undiagnosed physical condition, he/she may embark on a lifelong search for its physical cause. If, after seeing a medical specialist, the person decides that he/she suffers from migraine, an inherited physiological disorder without a known physical cause, he/she may accept the prevailing opinion that nothing medical can be done and just try to ignore the pain as best as possible. However, by consciously ignoring the bodily sensations leading to the pain, the individual is failing to utilize somatic information in an integrated fashion to prevent or to ameliorate future episodes of the disorder. How one interprets headache activity is very important, but what one does with the headache activity is even more important. The full integration of sensory information into consciousness is required to reverse the psychobiological processes leading to migraine onset and/or to reduce the likelihood of future episodes.

In this book I offer the concept of somatic awareness as the ultimate heuristic for achieving bodily well-being. A *heuristic* is generally defined as a device by which we understand something that is otherwise difficult to understand. Somatic awareness represents a heuristic because the experiential state of well-being to which I am referring is not easily described in psychological terms. It is also not readily defined in physiological terms. Although awareness of bodily events can lead to both positive and negative outcomes, my discussion of somatic awareness focuses on the positive or healing sensations. It is used to capture the experiential domain of bodily well-being. Somatic awareness is offered as the experiential counterpart of psychobiological healing processes within the individual.

The theoretical and clinical materials presented in this book adhere to the systemic framework I adopted in *Psychology and Health* (Bakal, 1992). The major tenets of systems models are that (1) systems are composed of interrelated parts, (2) no part of the system functions independently of the whole system, (3) change in one part is associated with change in all others, and (4) systems maintain a regular state of balance or homeostasis. In this volume, the focus or *searchlight* is on experiential bodily processes that can be used by the individual to maintain his/her health. Although I focus on bodily experience, I recognize that this experience occurs in the context of larger intrapersonal and interpersonal worldviews or systems. Somatic awareness, from my perspective, is an internal conscious referent that provides the individual with the means to make choices and lifestyle changes that can contribute to improving the health of his/her overall psychobiological system.

Somatic awareness represents the next stage in the evolution of holistic health care. Somatic awareness is not simply another form of alternative therapy. If anything, it stands in contrast to many of the alternative therapies in use today. Too often alternative techniques are promoted for their healing potential without due regard for the processes within the individual that he/she must activate for these treatments to be effective. Individuals still have a strong tendency to attribute illness and healing to factors external to themselves. Indeed, alternative medicine owes its popularity to this tendency. Yet much of the benefit from alternative practices occurs as a result of events within individuals themselves. Basic to achieving somatic awareness is the person's total experience of him/herself, which involves bodily sensations at the core. The bodily self is primary and occupies a place in consciousness that equals awareness of thoughts, feelings, and behaviors. Somatic awareness involves getting in touch with the somatic self for the purpose of improving physical health.

By encouraging individuals to shift their attention to healing experiences within themselves, we have the opportunity to develop a more systematic and responsible approach to holistic health. If we learn to listen and then work with body experience, we have the potential to change the very nature of medicine and health care at large. Somatic awareness, by directing attention to body experience, has the advantage of providing individuals with experiential access to healing processes within themselves.

My description of somatic awareness and its operation follows Sperry's (1987) concepts of the *emergent properties* of consciousness and *"top-down" determinism*. Rather than attempting to reduce human existence to some final common denominator, such as might be found in subatomic physics, Sperry proposed that we complement the natural science philosophy of examining control from below upward with a humanist–mentalist philosophy of examining control from above downward. For my purposes, the advantage of Sperry's conceptual framework lies in its integration of consciousness experience and natural science thinking. It allows reductionism and holism to live side by side. In adopting this approach, we need not reject the efforts of medical science to explain phenomena at lower or micro-levels. Rather, it is possible to view somatic awareness as an emergent property of the nervous system that can then exert causal control from above downward (Sperry, 1988). Somatic awareness as an emergent property within conscious experience is capable of influencing the bodily processes that determine its nature.

The balance of this chapter utilizes existing empirical evidence to illuminate the basic dynamic nature of somatic awareness. This evidence indicates that somatic awareness is far from being a passive state of the person. On the contrary, it is an active process that begins with volitional attention to the information coming from our bodies. How that information is used determines whether the individual experiences benefits or negative effects.

The remainder of this book reflects the potential of somatic awareness for increasing our ability to manage a diversity of common medical symptoms, to better understand the action and use of psychoactive and analgesic drugs, and to improve the mind–body interface in dealing with immunological disease conditions. Discussion of the healing power of somatic awareness with immune system illness is consistent with and supported by what is known about mind and immunity. Somatic awareness represents a universal guide for clinicians, researchers, and patients in directing the common pursuit of the medical, lifestyle, and psychobiological conditions that are likely to increase the strength of the immune system and maximize inner healing resources.

The book concludes with a discussion of common healing techniques that can be used to enhance and be enhanced by somatic awareness. Therapeutic touch, biofeedback, meditative awareness, and effortless breathing are presented as examples of techniques that professionals may use to strengthen somatic awareness in their patients. The therapeutic impact of these procedures can be increased by helping patients understand that they are simply aids to patient empowerment through somatic awareness development.

Many of the clinical examples in this book come from my own practice as a multidisciplinary team psychologist working in inpatient and outpatient programs within a hospital setting. Clinicians working in such settings are required to deal with a variety of problems and illness conditions, often within the same patient. The case examples come mainly from geriatric patients who often present with multiple symptoms, multiple disease conditions, and multiple drug dependencies. I have found that somatic awareness can often serve as a focus of treatment planning for the multidisciplinary team and that it provides patients with an understanding of their role in the process.

I first briefly trace the evolution of thought regarding the relevance of the perception of internal bodily events and then I explore research on the origins of bodily sensations. The key issues addressed are as follows:

1. The identification of somatic well-being in consciousness.
2. The physiological origins of internal bodily sensations.
3. Bodily sensations that accompany positive and negative emotional experiences.
4. Cognitive factors that determine whether bodily awareness is beneficial or counterproductive to health.

This chapter concludes with a discussion of somatic awareness in action for reducing migraine headache and for assisting in childbirth labor.

THE EVOLUTION OF IDEAS ABOUT BODY AWARENESS

Prior to the 19th century much was said about the special senses of vision, audition, taste, smell, and touch, but the insides of the body were considered to be "fairly insensible" (Boring, 1942). Philosophers and psychologists tended to ignore sensations arising from internal structures because there were no known internal sensors and sensations must normally have an external referent object, that is, something that can be seen, smelled, or touched. Descartes (1596–1650) made a distinction between perception of external worldly events and perception of internal bodily events, but his thinking on bodily perception received no serious attention—primarily because somatic awareness was not viewed as constituting a special or even a useful sense. Descartes is better remembered for his ideas on the dualistic nature of the mind and body which set the terms for the thinking that followed. The body experience in Western culture was ignored in large part because in Western philosophy since Plato's time the body has been viewed as the servant or vessel of the more "spiritual" mind:

> Modern Western man's thought and language has been strongly influenced by the dichotomy of psyche and soma implying the superiority of the intentional mind over the intentionless body. Dualistic thought restrains and circumscribes bodily perceptions and bodily awareness, it alienates "us" from our body: it is the mind thinking of the body rather than the body perceiving itself. (Ots, 1990, p. 22)

In 1826 Charles Bell presented a paper in which he proposed that muscles contain sensory as well as motor nerves and that these sensory nerves are the basis of a physical *sixth sense*. Weber, in 1846, used the term *Gemeingefuhl* to describe all internal bodily sensations (including pain) that were inaccessible to study through an external referent (Boring, 1942). In 1855 Alexander Bain, while reviewing the five special senses, spoke of a sixth sense that he referred to as *common* or *general sensibility*. Though he did not clearly specify the origins of this sense, he suggested that its source could be the muscles and nerves located throughout the peripheral nervous system. Bain was referring to a independent state of consciousness that provided awareness of internal biological activity. The general sense could be experienced in consciousness as a state of bodily ill-being or its opposite, bodily well-being. He felt that the cause of bodily ill-being was "nervous fatigue," the description of which resembles that of modern-day depression and/or chronic fatigue syndrome:

> The expression of the feeling is one of pain, not acute but deep seated and engrossing; collapsed features, restlessness, fretting, and melancholy. . . . The getting rid of life itself is one of the most natural desires when the condition assumes its most virulent forms. This is a proof of the total loss of freshness and tone throughout the entire substance of the nervous system, the final triumph of ennui. . . . The struggle that we maintain against painful inflictions of all kinds, whether bodily or mental, preys at last on the substance of the nervous system, and produces as its result this new form of evil. Hence the common source of complaint with all classes of sufferers—the weariness, the ennui, the heavy tread of time, the impatience, the impossibility of being effectually soothed or comforted. (pp. 124–125)

Bain's description of bodily well-being is vague but, like ill-being, is surmised to have a physical rather than a psychological origin. The state could be activated naturally or chemically and is experienced in consciousness as pleasurable and general but difficult to remember or describe when no longer present. Bain was referring to a bodily rather than to an emotional feeling.

There were others in Bain's era who spoke of a state of consciousness experienced as coexistence with our bodies—a state of *internal touch*. In 1884 Ribot asserted that the sense of the body, although usually vague and in the background of consciousness, constitutes the basis of human individuality or personality. According to Ribot, somatic awareness reflected the "*tone* of the sensory nerves, or the perception of the state of mean activity in which those nerves are constantly found, even in moments when they are not excited by external impressions" (p. 19). Ribot viewed body awareness as a fundamental feeling of existence that remained largely outside of awareness during periods of perfect health. This position suggested, contrary to my own, that awareness of the body is not a normal or a natural state of consciousness and that only comes to the fore during periods of illness. Ribot equated health with a state of psychological and physiological equilibrium that negated the need for the mind to be consciously aware of bodily activity. During periods of intense well-being or of illness, however, individuals became aware of their sensuous existence. Ribot clearly recognized that changes in the sense of the body contributed to dramatic changes in consciousness and personality, but he did not speculate on how the individual might use his/her sense of the body to attain or maintain health.

Dualistic thinking continued into the 20th century with the writings of Freud (1856–1939). In developing his structural/biological theory of the mind, Freud initially acknowledged the existence of somatic sensations. Later he decided that these sensations were best viewed as the raw material to which the mind's work is then applied (Sulloway, 1979). Freud began his career in the biological sciences but was ambivalent about pursuing a union between psychoanalysis and biology. He was defiantly opposed to contemporary physiological theories of mental events. He also believed that methods of controlling physical symptoms through conscious experience were of little value. For example, although he initially embraced hypnosis as a means of enhancing the patient's awareness of and control over bodily functions that had been lost due to hysterical paralysis, he eventually lost faith in hypnotic therapy. Consequently, in his theorizing, he began to probe for the presumed unconscious mental processes that he believed were ultimately responsible for unexplained physical symptoms. He became more interested in determining how the unconscious mind *worked on and transformed* incoming body information (e.g., in dreams) than in how patients use conscious somatic information to understand their physical selves. Consequently, the body in Freudian theory is definitely portrayed as a vessel of the mind.

But one of Freud's students, Sandor Ferenczi (Sulloway, 1979), saw the therapeutic potential of directly integrating bodily and mental dynamics. Ferenczi believed in trying to unravel psychological conflicts by encouraging patients to make changes in their bodily state. He realized, for example, that repressed memories could often be brought closer to consciousness by prompting patients to engage in a physical behavior antithetical to the repression of painful thoughts and feelings. In this way, he theorized, the body could be used to free the mind. One of his preferred strategies was to help patients achieve some degree of mind–body connectedness through the practice of physical relaxation during a psychoanalytic session. Such relaxation served to enhance conscious association by reducing psychological inhibitions.

The idea of reducing psychological inhibitions by releasing bodily tension was brought to prominence by one of Ferenczi's students, Wilhelm Reich (1942, 1962), an Austrian psychoanalyst with a gift for looking at the naked body and "reading" from it what impulses a person might be repressing through muscular contraction. In the tradition of early psychoanalytic theory, Reich focused his attention on repressed sexuality and developed a theory that, ultimately, orgasm is required to discharge excess musculoskeletal energy. Reich argued that energy not discharged through periodic orgasm may lead to bodily symptoms and personality attributes reflective of this failure. One such *biopersonality* pattern is characterized by shallow breathing and a stiffened belly combined with a character armoring in which thought processes are disconnected from bodily feelings. Orgasm was the recommended solution to this muscular and character armor—but not just ordinary orgasm. Orgasm for Reich was more of a mind–body sexual experience than most people have had, involving a full-body *plasmatic pulsation* of the embraced sexual partners—the objective not being orgasm per se but the total and completely free flow of energy between the partners.

The dynamic relationship between body tension and emotional suppression was brought into modern times with the writings of Alexander Lowen (1958). For Lowen, the motivating force of life was not sexual energy or libido but rather a fundamental *bioenergy* of the human body that manifests itself in psychological phenomena or somatic motion. Lowen realized that there was more to solving somatic problems than experiencing head-to-toe sexual orgasm. His broader objective during therapy sessions was to help patients learn to understand how tensions in various regions of their bodies were associated with repressed fears and hostilities. According to Lowen, a central objective of his approach was the *grounding* of patients in their legs and bodies. For Lowen, having a body sense of one's feet planted firmly on the ground equates with emotional and physical well-being. Since Lowen believed that body awareness is best achieved through body movement, he designed a number of exercises to increase patient perception of body parts and processes.

The 1960s initiated a shift in theorizing about the body. The body was no longer seen as a vehicle driven solely by the unconscious mind. Now a group of theorists and clinicians associated with humanistic psychology envisioned the body as potentially more conscious than unconscious (Otto, 1966). The human potentialities movement received its theoretical impetus from existential and humanistic philosophers who argued that human consciousness had potentials exceeding levels experienced during ordinary life. They recognized body experience as a key component of experiential growth and enlightenment. Awareness of the body was acknowledged as a positive state of mind and being. According to the theorists, a higher level of psychological wellness and spirituality is theoretically attainable by all.

Developing greater awareness of the body through movement (Feldenkrais, 1972) and touch (Pesso, 1969) were two popular techniques used to attain psychological growth. The Feldenkrais method uses nonstrenuous exercises designed to reeducate the nervous system and emphasizes learning from one's kinesthetic feedback. Pesso (1969) used body movement and physical touch during therapy sessions to make people more aware of their inner emotional dynamics. He began therapy sessions with an introduction to the "species stance," which requires participants to relax all their skeletal muscles "short of falling to the ground" (p. 6). The idea is to relax all voluntary muscles by letting the arms hang, allowing the head to drop, and letting the stomach protrude. Pesso made an observation that has since been noticed by all practitioners of body therapy: many people find it very difficult to let their body go in this fashion not because of fear of falling but because of fear of losing psychological control.

Thomas Hanna (1970) wrote about the healing and health potential of body consciousness. He offered the field of *somatics* as a means of studying bodily experience while at the same time transcending the mind–body distinction. Hanna believed that the body is experienced holistically, not in terms of specific sensations and/or symptoms. For Hanna, sensation is inseparable from perception and feeling. Hanna split consciousness into phenomenological and analytical modes. Somatics involves awareness of the inner body in phenomenological terms while perception of the external is represented in analytical consciousness. At this experiential level, as described by Hanna, it is possible to sense our physical selves and the external world without necessarily having to articulate these feelings in words. Hanna (1988) made a distinction between the objective body and the body as perceived in phenomenological consciousness:

> There are two ways in which a human being can be viewed: from the outside in, or from the inside out. Looked at from the outside, by a physiologist or a physician, human beings are very different from the beings they appear to be when they view themselves from the inside out. . . .
> What physiologists [and physicians] see from their externalized, third-person view is always a "body." What the individual sees from his or her internalized, first-person view is always a "soma." *Soma* is a Greek word that from Hesiod onward has meant "living body." This living, self-sensing, internalized perception of oneself is radically different from the externalized perception of what we call a "body." (p. 20)

There were other developments during the human potentialities period directed toward increasing the awareness of the body-self. The most important of these developments was the discovery of biofeedback. The promise of biofeedback as a means of attaining bodily insight and health reached a pinnacle during the late 1960s. In California, practitioners of biofeedback had discovered alpha-electroencephalographic (EEG) control as a nonchemical means to achieving mind enhancement and enlightenment. During this period, people speculated that biofeedback could be offered in university courses to enhance what was termed "physiological awareness." Students, it was thought, could be taught to appreciate the subjective experiences associated with their various physiological response systems.

Barbara Brown (1980) was an early proponent of the use of biofeedback for achieving health. In her book *Supermind: The Ultimate Energy* she marvels at both the ease and difficulty with which the human mind works with body information. She argued that once attention is directed toward the body, it becomes possible to sense a myriad of sensations that have significance for the health of the individual. She also recognized, however, just how difficult it is to initiate attention directed to the interior physical self. She noted that too often we do not perceive or act upon these sensations until they cause pain, and then it seems too late to do anything with the information:

> The first time I became aware of the power of unconscious thought was so dramatic I will never forget it. It happened on the final day of my first year in medical school. My mother had driven some five hundred miles to fetch me and my belongings back home, and there were only a few things to do before we left the medical complex. At lunch with some of my friends, we had gone through the cafeteria line delighted with the prospect of watercress and shrimp sandwiches and cold soup on that summer day. We sat at the table, and as I started to eat I suddenly became convulsed by an overwhelming nausea. Simultaneously I excused myself and ran hell-bent to the nearest restroom. With stomach in reverse peristalsis, and mouth filled with acid flow, I threw up just as I reached the closet basin. A bit later, white and weak, I rejoined my mother and my friends. I whispered to her what had happened, and she whispered back, "Is it because your grades are being posted now?" (Brown, 1980, p. 173)

Brown's experience captures the elusive nature of somatic awareness. It can be one of the most easily overlooked aspects of taking care of one's health. One reason it is so easy to overlook is that our language lacks words to express mind–body experiences. Other cultures have words that are closer to capturing the holistic essence of somatic awareness. In German, for example, there is the literary word *Leib,* which refers to both psychological and physiological well-being, although not necessarily in an integrated fashion. Chinese culture has the concept of *qi* (chi) or vital force, and the Chinese are culturally trained to experience their bodily *qi.*

Mindfulness is an Eastern mediation concept that has made its way into the holistic health literature. Mindfulness is compatible with but not identical to what I call somatic awareness. Mindfulness is central to Buddhism and refers to a clear, lucid quality of awareness regarding to the cognitive and emotional experiences of everyday life. Mindfulness or meditative awareness is a superordinate condition, a kind of universal awareness, a transcendence of our usual state of consciousness. Meditative awareness has three primary qualities: calmness, openness, and harmony. Somatic awareness from this perspective is limited because it ties consciousness to some "thing": sensation, feeling, or thought. With true meditative awareness, there is no need to "experience" the body, for it will take care of itself. Mindfulness, like meditation, deals with the totality of consciousness, and accompanying bodily changes are secondary. Complete meditative awareness has no "aware of" dimension—it does not contact anything. It is just perfectly aware. The bodily aspect of experience is there, because it is always there, but it doesn't receive attention.

With somatic awareness, the attention is directed to bodily experience—there is no need for an altered or unfamiliar state of consciousness, simply an awareness in consciousness of what is already there. The internal perception of bodily self and feelings of bodily well-being can be achieved without adopting a particular religion or philosophy of the universe. In trying to help elucidate the essence of somatic awareness, my editor suggested an analogy to the operation of a wheelbarrow:

> I imagine it sort of like a wheelbarrow. The wheel in front represents the somatic, bodily aspects of experience and carries the "load." The handles are the emotions and cognitions, which steer. It's much more effective to focus on where the front wheel is going and adjust direction through the handles, than it is to focus on the handles without paying much attention to where the front wheel is.

Generally our descriptions of bodily sensations rely on analogies with external objects or events. The sentence "I feel calm" uses a weather analogy. But analogies do not usually refer to characteristics of the internal state from which the sensations arose. It is not an easy matter to compare and share inner experiences with others. The difficulties in verbalizing inner experiences do not mean, however, that there are not commonalities to these experiences. After all, we do share the same neurophysiological structures that contribute to inner experiences.

THE SOURCE OF BODILY AWARENESS

What is it that we are aware of when we are somatically aware? We are aware of much more than the passive perception of internal bodily information. Somatic awareness is the experiential equivalent of an integrated psychobiological state. The nature of the experience is dynamic. Given that it is both psychobiological and dynamic in nature, it will prove difficult to identify its biological basis. Emotional, cognitive, social, cultural, and physiological factors are tightly bound in the experience.

Physiological Factors

Determining the physiological source of any bodily perception is far from straightforward. Sensations arising from the body are characteristically vague, hard to localize, and even harder to quantify. Internally, somatic sensations have their origins primarily in proprioceptive information coming from the muscles, tendons, and joints. Proprioceptive messages from skeletal and smooth muscle are carried through the dorsal-column medial-lemniscus system to the primary and secondary somatosensory cortex. This internal information is less specific than information from the external skin receptors involved with touch. But it is still capable of providing valuable information regarding body activity. The proprioceptive information coming from these muscles contributes to the somatic awareness experience, thereby making somatic awareness to a large extent a *muscle sense*. For example, we know that both skeletal muscle and smooth muscle are able to physiologically tense and relax.

Internal information from the viscera or internal organs (heart, lungs, vessels, stomach) also contributes to somatic sensations. Visceral information is more difficult to localize than information from the muscles, tendons, and joints. The internal organs located deep within the body transmit information to the brain through nonspecific pathways and terminate diffusely in higher brain centers. Receptors from body organs connect with multiple pathways. Visceral nerve fibers from the heart, for example, enter the spinal cord in multiple locations and link with fibers from other visceral areas. The net result is that sensations originating in the heart can be felt in areas away from the heart. An example of this, called "referred pain," commonly occurs during heart attacks, when damage to cardiac muscles can be perceived by the heart attack victim as pain in shoulders and arms rather than in the heart itself.

Research on perceptions from within the body has been restricted to observations based on selected physiological response system changes. This research has demonstrated that individuals are generally not very accurate in perceiving the status of their internal physiological responses. Such accuracy in perception can, however, improve with training and practice. Fisher (1986) reviewed a number of early studies

involving heart rate detection and found that, in the absence of training, individuals are able to estimate increases and decreases in heart
rate with no better than chance accuracy. With feedback, their performance improves but is not necessarily maintained outside the feedback
situation. Similar observations have been made concerning muscle tension, measured with surface electromyography (EMG). Although subjects are able to judge tension levels in various muscle groups, they generally cannot do much better than chance. But with training,
performance improves considerably, indicating that there is a potential
for recognition of body tension levels.

At this time there are no simple generalizations for determining
the degree to which individuals can correctly perceive bodily events.
Steptoe and Vögele (1992) presented volunteer female students with
three stress tasks involving mental arithmetic, mirror drawing, and
the cold pressor test and required the subjects to provide ratings of
bodily sensations experienced as "racing heart," "sweaty hands,"
"high blood pressure," and "shortness of breath." Heart rate, electrodermal activity, blood pressure, and respiration rate were recorded as
the corresponding physiological measures. The researchers found a
close association between the contour of responses in each physiological parameter and its corresponding sensation rating, and concluded
that the subjects were able to identify bodily sensations in a laboratory setting. The mean within-subject correlations were highest for
heart rate (.76), followed by systolic blood pressure/high blood pressure (.55), respiration rate/shortness of breath (.48), and skin con-
ductance/sweaty hands (.47). The researchers did, however, note
major differences in the accuracy of perception correlation coeffi-
cients across the 30 subjects. These differences were not due to differences in autonomic lability or measured trait anxiety. There was
no association between accuracy of somatic perception across the different physiological parameters. The researchers felt that their results
casts doubt on any general tendencies toward sensitivity and accuracy of somatic perception and on the notion that people vary on a
dimension of visceral sensitivity.

One disturbing finding of this research for the present thesis is
that subjects often base their judgment of physiological change on
their present level of anxiety and stress rather than on their objective
physiological state. Steptoe and Noll (1997) suggested that the positive
within-subject correlations between bodily perception ratings and
physiological measures reported by Steptoe and Vögele (1992) may
have been an artifact of the experimental procedure. Since, the ratings
were obtained during a series of mildly stressful tasks, the subjects may

have been making judgments based on what they believed should occur in such circumstance rather than on what actually did occur. To determine if this is what actually happened, Steptoe and Noll designed two tasks, viewing unpleasant slides of diseased skin and listening to an audiotape of a woman describing her discovery of skin cancer, which might be expected to cause physiological arousal but which in fact do not. Two additional tasks were also used. At the end of each task, subjects were asked to estimate their anxiety, stress, breathing, heart rates, and hand sweatiness. The researchers found that subjective ratings of bodily sensations mirrored ratings of anxiety and stress rather than objective physiological state; that is, subjective ratings of heart rate change reflected ratings of subjective anxiety and stress more than objective physiological change. The within-subject correlational data were very similar to the data reported by Steptoe and Vögele. There was a very wide variation from subject to subject in the correlations of bodily ratings and objective physiological activity. For example, the heart rate–heart rate rating correlations ranged from .95 to −.70 (a positive correlation indicates a close correspondence between fluctuations in objective physiological activity and perceptions of bodily state). The mean correlation between heart rate and ratings of variations in heart rate was .10 (near zero).

In summarizing the research data, there are two issues in need of clarification. First, somatic awareness is not reducible to the perception of fluctuations in specific internal organs or single response systems such as the heart rate or sweat gland activity (conscious life would be most disruptive if we were normally aware of each beat of the heart). Empirical studies of heart perception, although interesting, have little or no bearing on the state of somatic awareness. Somatic awareness has more to do with proprioception of skeletal and smooth muscle activity than of cardiac muscle activity. Second, we must accept the fact that bodily perception is often influenced by the situation or context in which it is occurring. As demonstrated in the Steptoe and Noll (1997) paper, people do base their perceptions of what is taking place internally on information other than what is actually taking place within their bodies. Beliefs of what "should occur" or what "might be occurring" are often stronger determinants of perceptions of bodily state than the actual bodily state itself. Although the decoupling of perceptions of bodily responses and objective responses is commonplace, it does not have to be the case. People can learn to use bodily information in an accurate and healthy fashion—especially if they are given guidance and encouragement in the use of such information.

Phantom "Body" Experience

In the final analysis bodily awareness is a conscious brain process. It is the brain that integrates and interprets incoming peripheral information against a background of its ongoing dynamic functions. Thus, in the search for peripheral determinants of bodily sensations, we cannot ignore the dynamic properties of the brain and the equally dynamic properties of the mind. The potential complexity of somatic awareness is evident from research dealing with phantom limb experiences. In these instances the awareness of a peripheral bodily sensation occurs in the physical absence of the actual body part. Phantom limb pain is the best known of these experiences. Approximately 70% of amputees experience burning, cramping, and other painful bodily sensations in the phantom limb following amputation. In many instances, these aversive bodily sensations continue for years following the limb removal. The source of these sensations is a mystery, but it is believed to involve both *central and peripheral* nervous system processes. Melzack (1990a) argued against explanations based on equating phantom sensations with peripheral nerve loss alone. There are occurrences of phantom sensations even when amputation has not occurred. He provided the example of patients who after being administered an anesthetic block of the nerves serving the arm temporarily experience a "third arm," usually at the side or over the chest. The phantom arm is unrelated to the position of the real arm when the eyes are closed but "jumps" into it when the patient looks at the arm. Also the descriptions given by amputees include reports of a full range of body sensations and feelings, including touch, pressure, warmth, sweatiness and fatigue. Paraplegics who suffer a break of the spinal cord and therefore have no somatic sensation below the break still report that they can "feel" their legs and lower body.

Melzack (1990a) also rejected explanations for phantom phenomena that are based on specific structures within the central nervous system (CNS). Surgical removal of areas within the somatosensory cortex fails to resolve phantom pain. Even more astonishing is his claim that a "substantial number of children who are born without all or part of a limb feel a vivid phantom of the missing part" (p. 90). He takes these observations as support for the existence of a partly innate, partly learned, neural network or *neuromatrix*. This neural network, he believes, is at the basis of one's physical self and presumably includes somatic awareness. The network is distributed throughout the brain and, although having a genetic component, acquires its individual identity or *neurosignature* through repeated activation. In this way, a particular neural network can evolve for phantom sensations.

Melzack's ideas, although speculative, serve as a reminder that the bodily sensations implicated in somatic awareness are not likely to have easily identified physiological substrates. Bodily sensations are often subtle and nondescript and their physiological underpinning will likely be equally subtle and nonspecific in origin. There may be a highly individualized somatic self that is based on an individual's total life mind–body experiences. Such ideas challenge the complexity rather than the veridicality of bodily sensations, so we need not delay using this dimension of consciousness to facilitate health.

Emotional Factors

Do specific emotions have a sensory component that contributes to the overall emotional experience? We usually think of emotional experience in terms of the external object of our emotion (e.g., loved ones). However, a hallmark characteristic of emotion is the bodily sensation felt. There may be a set of bodily sensations characterized by specific positive emotional states that, if identified, could be used to maximize the health and healing benefits of somatic awareness. The use of humor to manage cancer is a case in point. The benefits of humor may be accompanied by bodily sensations that are identifiable outside of humor episodes. I will examine this issue in detail. For now, I am interested in whether specific emotional feelings are associated with identifiable bodily sensations. There is only a small body of literature on the topic because few investigators have tried to measure the bodily sensations that accompany positive and negative emotional states.

Lyman and Waters (1986) asked college students to describe the bodily sensations they experienced during a large number of possible emotional states. Negative emotional states like anxiety, anger, and depression were associated with descriptors involving tension, tightness, weak/tired, burning, heaviness, and pain, whereas positive feeling states, like enthusiasm and joy, were associated with lightness, and others, such as love, friendliness, and feeling needed, were linked to warmth. Thus there is some evidence that identifiable classes of bodily sensations at least differentiate "bad" and "good" emotions. Bodily sensations of tension, tightness, and weakness are identifiable by patients with most disease states. Positive emotions were associated with sensations of lightness and warmth, which are readily generated by bodily relaxation. It is important to understand that bodily sensations, both negative and positive, can and do exist in the absence of specific emotional feelings. Thus, one can create sensations of bodily tension without feeling angry and one can create bodily warmth without receiving a good hug.

Several self-report questionnaires exist to assess body awareness correlates of negative feelings. These instruments tend to focus on the awareness of specific physical symptoms rather than general physical feeling states. The widely used Autonomic Perception Questionnaire (Mandler, Mandler, & Uviller, 1958), for example, asks respondents to indicate whether they feel hot, upset in the stomach, a lump in the throat, cold or chilly, and so forth when they are anxious or emotional. Similarly, the Private Body Consciousness Questionnaire (Miller, Murphy, & Buss, 1981) contains items reflecting bodily events associated with stress and tension. No effort is made to measure somatic awareness as a specific or general state of positive well-being.

Designing questionnaires to assess bodily awareness in the context of positive emotions is a needed next step. Today, we know much about negative feelings and body experience but very little about positive emotion and body experience. Shields, Mallory, and Simon (1989) developed an 18-item Body Awareness Questionnaire designed to assess what they called "attentiveness to normal bodily processes" rather than attentiveness to stressful bodily events. The questionnaire includes items referencing bodily cycles and rhythms ("I can tell when I go to bed how well I will sleep that night," "I notice specific body responses to changes in the weather") and the ability to detect small changes in normal physiological functioning ("I notice distinct body reactions when I am fatigued," "I know in advance when I'm getting the flu"). In a separate study Shields and Simon (1991) examined whether individuals who report a high degree of bodily awareness, as measured by the Autonomic Perception Questionnaire, during negative emotions, also evidence a high degree of nonemotional bodily awareness as measured by their questionnaire. This is an important issue since emotional and nonemotional bodily awareness are likely independent states of consciousness. Emotional symptoms are associated with strong autonomic responses (e.g., racing heart) and are quickly noticed without conscious effort. Attention to nonemotive bodily responses is different from emotional feeling in that it requires a form of *volitional attention* to conscious processes that are otherwise operating outside of awareness. Being aware of bodily sensations involved with strong emotional responses is not the same as being able to use bodily sensations to facilitate feelings of well-being. Supporting the distinction being made, the researchers found very low correlations between the two questionnaires, and concluded that nonemotional and emotional body awareness are different states of consciousness. Individuals who report volitional bodily experiences are not necessarily the same individuals who report nonvolitional bodily symptoms. The two categories of conscious experience occur independently.

Love and Empathic Support

Love and support from others are usually discussed as abstract concepts but feeling loved and cared for are powerful personal experiences with emotional, cognitive, *and* somatic components. People may not be aware of the somatic aspect of felt love, but it is very much there. A study from the Institute of HeartMath (McCraty, Atkinson, Tiller, Rein, & Watkins, 1995) is interesting in this regard. McCraty et al. reported that *self-induction* of a positive supportive emotional state was associated with the induction of smooth, even heart rhythms, defined in terms of reduced heart rate variability. The researchers developed a technique they called the freeze-frame method which instructs subjects to "consciously disengage from unpleasant mental and emotional problems, by shifting attention to the heart, . . . and [then] focus on sincerely feeling appreciation" (p. 1089). They demonstrated that the laboratory induction of *feelings of appreciation* were associated with power spectral density changes of the electrocardiogram (ECG) that were indicative of sympathovagal balance (reduced variability) or increased harmony of the sympathetic and parasympathetic innervations to the heart. By way of contrast, instructions to generate angry feelings resulted in a power spectral shift of the ECG to sympathetic dominance (increased variability). What is of particular interest is that the reductions in heart rate variability and presumed increase in cardiovascular health were associated specifically with feelings of appreciation and not just with any positive emotional feeling. Feeling appreciated obviously requires actions from other people to generate the feeling state.

Researchers have long recognized the positive power of social and family relationships in maintaining health and longevity. House, Landis, and Umberson (1988), for example, reviewed a number of prospective studies indicating that mortality is higher among socially isolated individuals. Russek and Schwartz (1997) presented data showing that measures of bodily feelings and warmth and psychological feelings of closeness with parents predicted health and illness some 35 years later. In the early 1950s, as part of the Harvard Mastery of Stress Study, a sample of healthy young college men were asked to describe their mother and father in terms of parental caring attributes (i.e., very close, warm and friendly, tolerant, strained). These same individuals were examined in midlife for the presence of diagnosed diseases. Individuals who as students had reported feelings of warmth and closeness with their mothers and fathers had far fewer diseases in midlife than individuals who during college perceived their parents to be low in warmth and closeness. Russek and Schwartz hypothesized that the perception of love may turn out to be "a core biopsychosocial–spiritual buffer, reducing the negative impact of stressors and pathogens and promoting immune functioning and healing" (p. 12). The notion that early experiences of love and caring from significant others is required to be able to self-soothe is basic to all developmental self theories. We will see, in the next chapter, how certain parental attachment patterns can facilitate or restrict an individual's ability to self-soothe.

The hypothesis that love and social support strengthen the individual's resistance to disease receives buttressing at the neuroendocrine level. Neuroendocrine regulation is a central facet of human physiological competence at any age and has been hypothesized to represent a critical pathway for the influence of "extrinsic" factors on patterns of health and aging. The hypothalamic–pituitary–adrenal (HPA) axis and sympathetic nervous system (SNS) together constitute a central neuroendocrine pathway that has a central role in maintaining ongoing, homeostatic regulatory processes of the body in the face of changing environmental stimuli. They also have known links to pathophysiological processes such as elevated blood pressure, serum cholesterol, and diabetes. This central pathway has been called a "superhighway" for both health and disease because it is involved in so many disease conditions (Kaplan, 1995).

One argument holds that the problem of all health and illness is essentially one of balance within the neuroendocrine system:

> Activation of these central regulatory systems is designed to mobilize energy stores and cardiovascular tone to facilitate cognitive and physical adaptation, which are crucial to survival. However, although activation of the HPA and SNS systems—with their accompanying elevations in glucocorticoids and associated increased serum glucose and lipids, immunosuppression, and increased cardiovascular tone—is indeed beneficial (and indeed frequently essential) in the short-term, such increased activation has also been linked to increased risks for many pathologies, such as cardiovascular disease, diabetes, hyperlipidemia, hypertension, and cancer, as well as immune function if activation is excessive or prolonged. (Seeman & McEwan, 1996, p. 460)

The term "allostatic load" has been used to describe the postulated link between neuroendocrine activity and health risks. As defined by McEwan and Stellar (1993), allostatic load refers to the "cumulative strain on the body produced by repeated ups and downs of physiologic response, as well as by the elevated activity of physiologic systems under challenge" (p. 2094), with this physiological activity being precipitated largely by our interactions with the world around us.

Social isolation and depression are known to have negative influences on this pathway. Studies have shown that the presence of a friend can decrease cardiovascular stress responses to laboratory stressors (Seeman & McEwan, 1996). The measurement of the meaning of the relationship is critical in predicting the outcomes of such studies. For example, studies have revealed that the presence of a "socially support-ive companion" may mean different things to men versus women. Kirschbaum, Klauer, Filipp, and Hellhammer (1995) demonstrated that the presence of a socially supportive companion (either a partner or a stranger) was associated with attenuated serum cortisol responses during the anticipatory period before a public speaking task only for men. With women, the presence of a partner was actually associated with a trend toward increased cortisol responses. Other studies (Seeman & McEwan, 1996) have found that the relationship between social support and reduced endocrine activity holds only for men. For women, evidence suggests that being with a partner can represent more of a need to take care of someone else rather than a need to be taken care of. This research indicates that women more often than men are turned to for help and that caring for others represents a "cost" of social relationships that is higher for women in terms of increased symptomatology and perceived stress. It would appear that women need to reevaluate their tendency to care for others, if it comes at a high cost to themselves.

Research is beginning to suggest that empathic relationships are more conducive to health than other forms of social support. This finding may have implications for somatic awareness, for empathy includes to some degree the ability to experience what another person is feeling at a bodily level. Somatic awareness may owe its developmen-tal existence in part to the ability to be empathically aware of the needs of others. Being able to "read" and support the feeling states of other individuals depends on having had conscious awareness of similar feel-ings within oneself. Uchino, Cacioppo, and Kiecolt-Glaser (1996) dem-onstrated that the same physiological symptoms and diseases that respond positively to somatic awareness interventions also respond pos-itively to the presence of empathic social support. Thus self-controling somatic awareness strategies like meditation and relaxation seem to yield similar physiological events within the person as a loving and/or caring relationship.

In exploring the mediators of social support on the immune sys-tem, Uchino et al. (1996) stated that the associations between social support and immune function are significant even when controlling for behavioral health practices, such as diet and exercise. They noted that stress and depression have reliable effects on immune function and that part of the association between social support and immune function is mediated by these factors. However, they also stated that others have found that life events, depression, and anxiety levels *are not the key factors* responsible for the association between social support and immune function. Therefore, although health-related behaviors, depression, and life stress have effects on aspects of immune function, these factors do not appear to be the major pathways explaining the associations between social support and immune function. What this suggests is that there is some as yet undiscovered healing influence associated with empathic/emotional interactions. I believe that the healing influence is based in a universal need for soothing from others and that the sensory components of this need are identifiable and reproducible in consciousness.

Generally, the need for care from others as well as the accompanying positive sensory state operates outside an individual's consciousness. Consequently, we can never be certain if the need and its sensory benefits were actually activated and realized in studies investigating the health benefits of social support. An example of such a research study is provided by Levine et al. (1979). They trained family members to provide support regarding management of a patient's hypertensive state. The support was instrumental rather than empathic in delivery: a trained community interviewer provided the patient's spouse with ways to deal with the patient's knowledge, attitudes, and behaviors concerning hypertension and its management. The results indicated that family support was able to decrease diastolic blood pressure below the limits for hypertension. I cannot determine from the study's description whether the benefits were largely educational (i.e., better medical adherence) in nature, or, as I suspect, the result of a husband and wife working together to improve their relationship and caring for one another.

The link between emotional support and improved health must in some way be connected to the naturally soothing effects of supportive others. At the psychological level, social support may reduce perceptions of stress and feelings of loneliness, depression, and other negative emotional feelings. Laboratory studies suggest that the higher cardiovascular reactivity seen in situations involving low social support may translate to gradual elevations in tonic blood pressure across the lifespan. Exposure to situations involving lack of caring and hostility in the form of racial discrimination, for example, is hypothesized to explain the twofold greater prevalence of tonic hypertension among the U.S. black population than among the U.S. white population (Krieger & Sidney, 1996). For many blacks, living in a white-dominated society may necessitate very close control of their feelings and limit both emotional and somatic awareness within themselves. The same analysis would apply to any disadvantaged group in our society.

This discussion of emotion and social support awareness indicates the need for a systemic and integrated approach to somatic awareness. Somatic awareness has significant health and healing potential but its understanding and application must be undertaken in the context of the individual's emotional and interpersonal lifestyle. The systemic nature of somatic awareness will become even more apparent in the next section, where I examine how beliefs, attitudes, and attributions influence the perception of bodily sensations.

Cognitive Factors

Cioffi (1991) stressed the significance of a person's interpretation of a bodily event in determining the course of that event. This is an extremely important point: cognitive interpretation or attribution is a part of understanding all bodily experience. This means that all aspects of the human psyche, including past experience, unconscious mechanisms, beliefs, and attitudes, as well as the situational context of the bodily response, may influence how we perceive bodily sensations in consciousness. This is why health professionals are often unwilling to accept the accuracy of patient-reported bodily experiences unless the report is accompanied by some biological or physiological evidence. Clinicians working in the field of pain understand very well that the pain experience consists of more than a pure sensation: it includes a significant cognitive component. Although the sensory component of pain captures its intensity and quality, the cognitive components reflects the person's emotional reactions to the pain and his/her fears about what the pain means. Melzack (1990b) hypothesized that there may be different CNS pathways mediating the sensory and cognitive aspects of pain.

Whenever there is pain, the magnitude of the response to that pain is heavily influenced by the situation in which the person is experiencing the pain. The relationship between situational context and pain is demonstrated in a classic study by Beecher (1959). Beecher examined pain reports and the pain medication requests of injured soldiers and found that their noncombat injuries were perceived as more painful than the injuries they incurred during combat. He reasoned that combat-related injuries were perceived as less painful, presumably because they enabled the soldiers to leave battle. Civilian injuries, on the other hand were associated with different fears, such as loss of family, loss of life, and so on. Beecher's work has been used to demonstrate the power that the meaning given to a sensory stimulus has in the activation of the emotional component of the pain system. The fact that no isomorphic (one-to-one) relationship exists between pain report and injury has led to a definition of pain as a subjective, perceptual experience with both sensory and affective qualities.

Less dramatic examples of Beecher's observations are common in clinical practice.

> I was recently asked to see an 84-year-old patient who was admitted to hospital with excruciating and debilitating back pain. He was no longer able to function independently at home. Image scans revealed significant osteoporosis and deterioration of his spine. A call to his son revealed another picture. Apparently this patient had one remaining passion in life: model train building. Indeed, during the clinical interview, he was quite animated when he showed me photographs of a very extensive model train set. He revealed no evidence of pain during this period. The patient's son confirmed that his father's pain was highly selective or situation-specific. "When I ask Dad to visit and spend time with myself and the grandchildren he is often grimacing, suffering, and in too much pain to participate in family activities. But when someone visits him and expresses an interest in his hobby, he is scrambling under tables, connecting and disconnecting wires and showing little or no pain. It is hard to believe that he is in as much pain as he claims."

Social psychologists have repeatedly shown that by manipulating situational context cues, they can confuse individuals into misreading bodily information (Schachter & Singer, 1962). Although this research increased understanding of the presence of contextual/environmental information in interpreting bodily information, it has also had the unfortunate impact of trivializing the theoretical significance of actual bodily events taking place beneath the skin. A number of experiments have used falsified feedback to show that the cognitive information provided about bodily events can override the direct perception of physiological events themselves in determining a subject's understanding of what is taking place within the body. Valins (1967) went so far as to state that nonveridical cognitive representations of physiological events should have the same effects as veridical ones. That is, it does not matter whether the perception of bodily change is accompanied by actual bodily change, as long as the person believes that bodily change has taken place. Valins tested this hypothesis by exposing male subjects to slides of nude women. While they viewed the slides, they listened to tape-recorded clicks which they had been misled into believing represented their heart rates. Apparently, the subjects gave higher attractiveness ratings to slides they believed were associated with increased heart rates. Similar experiments using placebo study designs have demonstrated that subjects could readily be persuaded to experience sensations without the obvious bodily counterpart, such as feeling sensations of excitement when they are physiologically calm or sensations of an elevated blood alcohol level even though their alcohol intake has been minimal. Such social psychological research has had a negative effect on understanding of the significance of bodily experience for issues of health and illness. By giving primacy to cognition to the exclusion of bodily sensation, the social psychological approach has contributed to a general distrust of bodily information. This distrust has reinforced notions that there is no useful information coming from the body.

On the positive side, the social psychological model has emphasized the power of cognitive meaning in determining how we interpret, react to, and ultimately experience our bodies. Cioffi (1991) presented a very strong argument for viewing bodily experiences as being determined by cognitive–perceptual processes, distinct from actual sensory-physiological events. Her thesis is that physical symptoms are heavily influenced by socially influenced interpretations: people "act on their *internal* representations of their illness and of their symptoms; that is, they respond to their private, subjective, sometimes idiosyncratic world of interrelated beliefs, fears, competencies and goals" (p. 26). Cioffi reminds us that physical symptoms are subject to complex cognitive processes, and therefore are susceptible to influences beyond those explained by physiological mechanisms alone.

Cioffi (1991) provided an everyday example of the different cognitive–perceptual processes that may take place in reading one's body during exercise:

> While bicycling to the office, my hand temperature drops 0.5 degrees (the objective *physical state*). If I am obsessing about the lecture I must give, or if my route is marked by potholes, or if an old knee injury is acting up, I may never notice the mild physiological change in my hand; the competition for my fixed attentional capacities is, in this case, among several compelling internal and external events. But suppose that both my mind and my path are clear of competing clutter. I will most likely become aware of the physical sensation of cold hands, and this basic *somatic label* is now part of my attentional field.
>
> Once it is noticed, I will almost invariably *attribute* the sensation to something. If I believe that my hands are cold because my circulation is bad, then the sensation becomes a symptom-evidence that something is

wrong with me. I could arrive at this symptomatological attribution in one of two ways. First, the sensation of cold hands could confirm a pre-existing belief ("I've suspected I have poor circulation, and this is further proof"). Indeed, if I had been worrying about my health before beginning my commute, I would be actively searching for information that had a plausible bearing on this concern. In this case, a *pre-existing hypothesis* about my health affects both my awareness of and my attribution for the sensation. Alternatively, the perceived physical sensation could become the event for which an attributional search is launched. In either case, my sketchy self-diagnosis will include the consequences that I imagine are possible outcomes to my hypothesized malady.

My attribution for the sensation need not be symptomatological, however. If I believe that my cold hands are a normal response to the fall chill in the air, the somatic label will not be interpreted as a symptom, as the word is usually understood. Rather, it will be viewed as an appropriate physiological response to the external environment. Likewise, I could believe that all my blood has gone to my hard-working leg muscles, and thus I would be making an attribution that supports a hypothesis of fitness.

Even given a fixed somatic perception and an attribution for it (i.e., "my hands are cold, and it is due to poor circulation") my *behavioral* (and psychological) response to this construal will also depend on the *mediators of thought and action*, such as my mood, my coping repertoire and choices, and my general and situation-specific goals. For example, I may choose (or be prone) to respond to the threat of illness by actively distracting myself, or I may be compelled to do so today because of the importance of the upcoming lecture. (p. 30)

There is no question that attribution is a powerful process in medicine. An illness attribution often leads people to selectively search for sensations associated with that illness and to interpret incoming sensory information relative to it. Biomedical disease attributions in particular can limit or preempt opportunities for patients to utilize somatic awareness to control their condition. For example, when patients attribute their fibromyalgia or arthritic pain to an exclusively biological process, they tend to believe that the symptom is beyond their control. After all, they reason, if it is a biomedical disease, then it is not "all in their head." Once this attribution is made, it can be extremely difficult to use somatic awareness in a therapeutic manner without some change in their attribution.

Although cognitions and disease are independent events at one level of analysis, they are highly interrelated events at another level of analysis. Within the psychobiological framework, psychological, physiological, and psychobiological processes are linked to each other (Bakal, 1992). Disease processes and illness behaviors, as well as health behaviors, are interdependent. Illness behavior concepts may point to differences in coping, but a psychobiological approach is required to explain the pathways through which behavior is able to prevent illness and maximize health. Central to understanding the term "psychobiology" is the appreciation of a persons' total awareness or experience of themselves, involving thought, feeling, and bodily sensations:

> Whether we are dealing with emotional conditions involving anxiety or depression, stress, chronic pain disorders, or life-threatening disease, we are seeking to identify very subtle experiences within persons which can be tapped directly and indirectly to provide a [significant] degree of personal symptom management and improve health. In effect, we are speaking of individual awareness of the integration or union of a person's thoughts, feelings, sensations, and bodily reactions. Many factors impede awareness of this state but its importance in maintaining health in a complex world is without question. (Bakal, 1992, p. 7)

Adoption of somatic awareness as a health promotion strategy will be greatly enhanced with improved understanding of the psychobiological determinants of different illness conditions. As long as illnesses such as fibromyalgia and arthritis remain understood solely as biochemical disease conditions, we can expect sufferers to continue to exhibit beliefs and coping strategies that are potentially maladaptive. By shifting cognitive attributions of patients to include psychobiological determinants beyond biochemistry per se, it will become possible to have them understand that the biological substrate of their affliction is also a condition that is inextricably tied to their thoughts, feelings, and bodily sensations. Only then will it become possible to help them understand that their role in contributing to illness recovery is best achieved by developing enduring and overriding habits of somatic awareness.

Fear of Bodily Awareness

Many professionals view the link between bodily awareness and health in negative terms: the more attention paid to the body (usually a symptom), the worse the health. Awareness of the body is seen as a function of poor health or overconcern with health. Physicians and therapists often tell their patients to ignore bodily symptoms in the hope that the intrusiveness of the symptom will be reduced. Paying attention to one's body is viewed as a sign of moral weakness or indicative of a psychiatric condition such as hypochondriasis.

Psychological research with chronic disease conditions is often conducted with the aim of supporting the "not thinking about the body" perspective. Hansell and Mechanic (1991) found, for example, that elderly individuals who think about their bodies are also more likely to think about and report more physical symptoms over the course of a year than individuals who devote less conscious attention to their bodies. They assessed bodily awareness by asking a sample of older adults, during a personal interview, whether they ever think about how their body feels, focus on how it works, or wonder about why it feels the way it does. They also asked questions about perceived health status and number of reported physical illnesses. The majority of subjects were interviewed twice, with each interview separated by a 12-month interval. Hansell and Mechanic found a positive correlation between level of reported bodily awareness and longitudinal decreases in self-assessed health, suggesting that heightened bodily awareness is a negative attribute and that it not only leads to poorly perceived health but also to excess use of the health care system. Many similar studies have found that increased attention toward the body seems to lead to increased symptom reporting and poorer reports of health. However, these studies are dealing only with individuals who are aware of their bodies from an illness or sickness perspective. No one has considered that bodily sensations in the form of somatic awareness might be used to improve and maintain good health.

The fear of personal information, bodily or otherwise, is embedded in our cultural psyches. Some years ago Eric Cassell (1976) published a paper with the title "Disease as an 'It.'" He provided examples of how patients talk about their diseases and symptoms as "Its," as foreign objects apart from themselves. One example involved a woman who, prior to developing swelling and pain in her knees, described her knees as "nice" and as a positive part of her physical being. When they became swollen and painful, she referred to her knees as an *it* that was very swollen and fat. Many other symptoms are depersonalized in speech and action in a similar fashion. Migraine sufferers often refer to their condition as "it" ("Why is *it* happening now?", "I wish *it* would leave me"). Even anxiety symptoms are dissociated in this manner. Patients experiencing a panic episode will describe "waiting for *it* to pass" in the same terms as a fever experience. It is very common for diseases and symptoms not to be felt as part of the patient's personal body experience.

There is a school of thought in psychology that believes that any form of self-directed attention results in negative psychological experiences. These theorists believe that self-focused attention retards the process of self-delusion that is required for normal living (Gibbons, 1991). This line of thought had its origins in the body image research of Wolff in the 1930s (Wicklund, 1991). Wolff published a series of studies showing that subjects often had difficulty recognizing their own voices from audio playbacks or their profiles/body parts from drawings. Wolff concluded that personal information presented in this way forces individuals to realize discrepancies in how they "should" sound or look relative to internal standards associated with the ideal self. Focusing attention on the self activates a self-evaluation process whereby the individual compares him/herself with an internalized societal standard that he or she holds on that self attribute. Since these standards are usually beyond reach, self-awareness represents an unpleasant or aversive state (Duval & Wicklund, 1972). A disposition toward chronic self-focus has been linked to chronic negative affect, including both anxiety and depression.

Some self theorists take an extremely pessimistic view of the human potential for health through introspection. Self-focused attention, in their view, is inherently associated with anxiety. Terror management theory (Pyszczynski, Greenberg, Solomon, & Hamilton, 1991) holds that self-awareness is a curse of humankind. According to Pyszczynski et al., self-awareness is the innate ability to become aware of "the tenuous nature of existence, of the ever-present potential for pain and injury, and, most importantly, of the inevitability and unavoidability of death" (p. 71). They argue that "this awareness of our vulnerability and mortality gives rise to the potential for paralyzing terror" (p. 71). According to the theory, it is our cultural worldview that protects us from the existential reality of death: our culture provides each individual with a role through which he or she can view him/herself as valuable or useful. This sense of value is the basis of self-esteem and protects the individual against the anxiety that can be caused by awareness of our limited time on earth.

Fear of existential reality might impede an individual's perception of body self. There are instances, for example, when fear or avoidance of body sensations may originate in part from conscious or unconscious fears of the psychological self. Elderly patients with somatic symptoms, for example, do not like to think about themselves on any level and prefer to "keep busy" or "keep their thoughts on something other than themselves." Is the desire to maintain an external focus due to some unconscious existential fear of inevitable death, as suggested by terror management theory, or is it simply due to lifelong coping styles associated with avoidance of bodily information? Many of our present elderly population were raised with an ethic of working hard and not "wasting time" thinking of their own bodily needs. An illustration of how lifelong commitment to a work ethic might reveal itself in late-life symptoms is provided in the following case:

A 78-year-old patient complained of being unable to nap in the daytime or sleep throughout the night although he was in a state of exhaustion. He had no difficulty falling asleep, but once asleep he would awaken in a few minutes in a state of extreme panic and remain agitated for hours if not days. The panic state and associated symptoms were extremely frightening, to the extent that he preferred to stay as busy as possible in order to avoid thinking about himself or falling asleep. The clinical issue was whether his fear of sleep and associated symptoms were the result of existential issues, coping styles, or both. He had worked extremely hard throughout his life and he could never accept resting or taking a nap during the day. He considered rest a sign of laziness or weakness. In his younger days as president and owner of a large company, he remained afraid to nap in his office for "fear of being caught." If he happened to inadvertently fall asleep, he would waken with an extreme startle. The patient also dreaded the beginning of each day and feared the thought of being by himself without something meaningful to do. His present fear of sleeping during the day had its behavioral beginnings during his working days. It may, however, also have an existential component as well because he was constantly afraid of not doing something useful or worthwhile from morning to night. The cultural worldview has not provided retired individuals the means to conceive of themselves as worthwhile.

Not thinking about or fearing the body reflects cultural norms that can be modified. There is no a priori reason why bodily attention should be indicative of personal weakness or threatening in nature. The body has much to teach in terms of healthy living—we only have to listen to it.

SOMATIC AWARENESS AND ASYMPTOMATIC DISEASE

Medical conditions vary enormously in terms of the sensory information that accompany changes in underlying pathophysiology. The example of migraine presented earlier illustrated a symptom condition that is associated with considerable bodily information that can be used to regulate the disorder. Other symptom conditions, however, provide individuals with far less specific sensory information or none at all. Hypertension is an example of such a medical condition. Hypertension is often described as a "silent killer" because of the common belief that hypertensive individuals are unable to detect severe elevations in their blood pressure. Many hypertensives, however, do believe that they can tell when their blood pressure is elevated and when it has returned to normal. In making this judgment, they usually make reference to bodily sensations that occur with experiences of anxiety and stress, even though they may or may not report feeling subjectively anxious or distressed. For example, hypertensive-prone patients often state that they suspect that their blood pressure is elevated when they feel out of breath. They may or may not understand why they are experiencing breathlessness.

We need to know, then, if hypertensive individuals intuitively know when their blood pressure is elevated, what is the nature of the bodily information these individuals are experiencing in relation to their blood pressure increases? This would constitute a necessary first step in the development of reliable somatic awareness strategies for blood pressure regulation. At the moment, relaxation strategies have not been associated with stable improvements in clinically elevated blood pressure. Some subjects report reductions in blood pressure following relaxation training while others do not. These studies were not designed to increase somatic awareness per se. Therefore it is unknown whether the individuals participating in such projects understood the importance of integrating the somatic experiences of isolated relaxation training with the somatic experiences of daily living. I suspect that they did not, and consequently it is less than surprising to learn that the occasional practice of relaxation had little or no impact on long-term blood pressure readings. However, the observation that temporary reductions occurred is extremely encouraging, as it suggests that the longer term practice of somatic awareness by individuals susceptible to hypertension would result in stable reductions in their blood pressure.

There is surprisingly little research examining whether patients are aware of significant increases in their blood pressure. A study by Baumann and Leventhal (1985) is one of a handful that have examined this question. The study involved 44 employees of an insurance company who agreed to monitor their blood pressure twice daily for a 2-week period. Prior to each reading, subjects were asked to make a prediction as to whether the blood pressure reading would be higher, the same, or lower than the previous reading. Subjects also completed checklists that assessed moods, for example, angry, sad, afraid, and energetic, and symptoms such as flushed face, shortness of breath, sweaty palms, and dizziness. These moods and symptoms have been found to be predictive of blood pressure levels in other research. Overall the subjects were poor predictors of blood pressure changes, although some subjects were better than others. The authors found stronger associations between reported moods/symptoms and blood pressure *predictions* than between moods/symptoms and *actual* blood pressure changes, suggesting to them that subjects are relying more on social stereotypes of what "should" predict blood pressure changes than what actually does predict such change. They worried that people with elevated blood pressure may be relying on inaccurate information and inappropriate self-treatment by using mood and unrelated somatic symptoms. Baumann and Leventhal's study may not have been a fair test of the ability of hypertensives to detect internal blood pressure levels as the subjects were largely normotensive and did not show significant variability in their pressure variations in their readings on a day-to-day basis.

The question as to whether it is possible for hypertensive individuals to accurately perceive elevations in their blood pressure cannot be scientifically answered at this time. Clinically, however, I have seen a number of patients who know when their blood pressure is elevated and what they need to do to return the pressure to normal. Pennebaker and Watson (1988) demonstrated that hypertensive individuals are able to show some accuracy (i.e., greater than chance) in predicting blood pressure elevations in response to a variety of laboratory provocations. Still, Pennebaker and Watson believe that it may not be possible to identify sensations and/or symptoms that are directly indicative of hypertension. They suggest that such bodily cues need not be available if the hypertensive individual can identify *other sensations and feelings* that correlate with elevations and reductions in blood pressure. In their study Pennebaker and Watson examined the relationship of several bodily symptoms (sweaty hands, tense stomach, fast pulse, warm or hot body, headache) and feeling states (annoyed or angry, tense, excited, frustrated rushed) *thought to be* correlated with elevated blood pressure. These symptoms and feelings correlated with changes in blood pressure but the correlations were highly idiosyncratic for each subject. Indeed, in some subjects the correlations were in the opposite direction. Fast pulse and warm body were the sensations reported by the greatest number of subjects to correlate with increases in systolic blood pressure. Another frequently reported sensation was breathlessness. Excited and tense were the feeling states most frequently reported.

Through these intrasubject correlations Pennebaker and Watson were able to provide some empirical support for the hypothesis that direct awareness of the bodily response underlying hypertension need not be perceived if a consistent sensory correlate of the bodily response is perceptible. While it may not be feasible to train individuals to become more sensitive to actual blood pressure elevations, it is possible to increase individual awareness of specific and/or nonspecific somatic sensations that are reliably related to decreases in blood pressure. The fact that the link between blood pressure elevation and the correlated perceived symptom is highly idiosyncratic indicates that self-regulation strategies might need to be individually tailored.

The studies by Baumann and Leventhal and Pennebaker and Watson are important for directing attention toward recognition of cues associated with elevated blood pressure. Similar isolated studies exist for diabetes, with research showing that non-insulin-dependent diabetic individuals are also able to indirectly detect hyperglycemia and hypoglycemia by relying on sensations such as dizziness and light-headedness within themselves (Diamond, Massey, & Covey, 1989). As with hypertensives, the level of bodily detection observed in these studies varied enormously from subject to subject, but the evidence suggests the potential for greater use of somatic awareness is present across these two disease conditions. The hypertension and diabetes awareness studies indicate that it might be feasible to continue the search for experiential bodily correlates of both hypertension and diabetes. Somatic awareness could then be used to maximize the individual's chances of management of these disease conditions.

Many other medical disease conditions provide the individual with no obvious sensory information that can be utilized to directly manage the underlying disease processes. This topic has received so little research attention that at this time we cannot be certain what sensory information might accompany various disease processes and conversely what somatic information might be used to reverse these processes. There is a need for a phenomenological physiology that would reveal to us how we experience our bodies from living inside them.

In the balance of this chapter, I take a detailed look at two conditions that do provide sensory information to patients: migraine headache and childbirth labor. Both conditions illustrate the health potential of somatic awareness.

THE MANAGEMENT OF MIGRAINE

With psychophysiological disorders such as migraine headache, the sufferer is often able to identify sensory information early in the developing symptom episode that can then be used to abort at least lessen the severity of the attack. The use of bodily sensations to prevent the developing migraine episode is an excellent example of somatic awareness in practice.

Headache is the most frequently occurring pain symptom in the population, with 1-year prevalence estimates for migraine ranging from 10% to 20% and corresponding prevalence estimates for tension-type headaches ranging from 30% to 80%. Although the majority of these individuals experience less than one headache per month, a sizable number experience headache on a regular basis. There is a also a subgroup of patients who experience migraine and tension-type symptoms on a daily or near-daily basis; these individuals are extremely difficult to treat (Bakal, Demjen, & Duckro, 1994).

The dominant theories of migraine argue that it is primarily neurological or vascular in nature (Blau, 1990). Recently, there has been increasing acceptance of a psychobiological explanation for migraine (Bakal, 1982; Bakal et al., 1994). In spite of publicized claims for the effectiveness of a wide number of alternative therapies, drug control remains the treatment of choice for most headache sufferers. Migraine still tends to be analyzed and managed from a biomedical model. All the evidence suggests, however, that migraine susceptibility can be greatly reduced by having sufferers attend to bodily signs and symptoms indicative of an impending headache episode.

Attention to Early Warning Signs

An amazing number of migraine headache sufferers complain of persistent tightness in the neck and shoulder region. The prevalence of neck symptoms in migraine was first recognized by Harold Wolff (1937), the founder of modern migraine research. Wolff also noticed that the majority of his migraine patients were seldom pain-free outside of the migraine attack:

> There is another type of head pain which occurs in migraine patients. It may be present concomitantly or in the interval between migraine attacks. Such headache is nonpulsatile, of low or moderate intensity, and may last for days, weeks, or years. The individual feels as if he has a hat on when he has none; that his neck is in a cast; that his shoulders are sore; that if he could be rubbed he would feel more comfortable. (p. 1503)

Wolff clearly recognized the presence of nonpainful and painful sensations outside the actual migraine attack, but he did not view these persistent low-grade sensations/symptoms as having import for understanding the etiology of the more dramatic symptoms of the migraine episode or how these symptoms might be utilized by the migraineur to abort the actual migraine attack and reduce overall migraine susceptibility. Other early warning symptoms experienced by migraineurs include pallor, dizziness, aching muscles, and paresthesias (Amery, Waelkens, & Vandenbergh, 1986).

The first signs of migraine headache activity or the dull headache activity between migraine episodes are seldom perceived by headache sufferers as having coping value. They are more likely to be interpreted as meaning that one must prepare for another episode of pain, sickness, and disappointment. Better to ignore the worsening symptoms, migraineurs say, and get on with the day as long as one can. Therefore, somatic sensations are generally ignored by the sufferer in the hope that the condition will disappear or that as much as possible can be accomplished before the pain becomes unbearable.

This avoidance of sensory information by the migraine sufferer is related to the pattern of headache-related thoughts that occur before and during headache attacks. The more severe the attacks, the more they engage in nonadaptive headache-related thoughts (Bakal et al., 1994). For most headache victims, avoiding the underlying sensory symptoms and putting on a "brave face" seems to be the only alternative. Many patients actively avoid attending to their bodies out of fear that their symptoms will become worse. Moreover, many physicians encourage migraine patients to ignore benign bodily symptoms and get on with living. However, cognitive avoidance is not my recommended strategy for managing pain or any other bodily symptom.

Successful migraine management is based on *awareness* of rather than *avoidance* of bodily function. This point is seldom appreciated. Some of the most widely employed and *least successful* coping strategies used by headache sufferers (as well as other pain patients) include diverting attention, employing positive self-statements, ignoring pain, praying, increasing activity, and reinterpreting the pain (i.e., imagining something that is inconsistent with the experience of pain). Many of these strategies are characterized by an attempt at avoidance of the underlying pain. Research suggests that the more avoidance strategies are used, the longer the pain lasts (Bakal et al., 1994).

I have witnessed countless migraineurs who attempt to struggle through a migraine by ignoring the pain the best they can and muddling on with the day's demands. But avoidance of pain is psychologically exhausting, physiologically taxing, and usually results in a worsening of the symptom. The *weekend migraine* is the best clinical example of this style of coping and outcome. Individuals susceptible to this type of migraine function throughout the work week *in spite of* a low-grade headache but as soon as the weekend comes they experience a severe debilitating rebound form of migraine pain.

Coping behaviors for dealing with pain and other symptoms are successful to the extent that they result in recovery from the pathophys-

iological processes responsible for the migraine pain. Volitional attention to body response is a key factor in helping this happen. The difficulty with cognitive coping strategies involving positive self-talk and/or
avoidance is that such strategies divorce the individual from the psychobiological processes underlying the headache. The issue is not one
of unidirectional attention toward or avoidance of pain. Rather, it is
one of attending to the body's response to a given strategy. If one
directs attention away from the pain and this results in a recovery from
the underlying headache mechanisms, then the strategy is effective.
However, similar distraction may not be effective during the next headache episode. The individual may need to lie quietly and focus on
attending to and reducing the actual pain sensations. Both attention
outward (e.g., listening to soothing room sounds) and attention inward
(e.g., monitoring slow and regular breaths) can be used in a complementary manner to lessen pain and restore normal physiological function.

The goal behind somatic awareness is symptom attenuation rather
than symptom elimination. The key to self-regulation is becoming
more rather than less aware of body sensations that accompany
thoughts, feelings, and behavior. The approach is difficult, since many
patients lack the proclivity to look inward. It is especially difficult for
them to grasp the distinction between preoccupation with their symptoms as somatization and their bodily reactions as somatic awareness.

Although the concept of somatic awareness often does not find its
way into the conscious treatment plan for migraine headache, it is not a
completely novel concept historically. It seems to be better understood
in sports psychology, where athletes have long recognized the power of
somatic awareness to enhance performance. Morgan and Pollack
(1977) reported years ago that elite marathon runners, when compared
to their less experienced counterparts, were more likely to use a form
of somatic awareness in dealing with the sensations generated by running. The less experienced runners were more likely to use cognitive
strategies that had no relation to the sensory experiences of running,
such as recalling early experiences, working mathematical exercises,
and hearing favorite music. These strategies were also accompanied by
efforts to "run or fight through" the pain when it became noticeable,
which led to increased discomfort, pain, and discouragement. The cognitive strategies used by inexperienced runners resemble those
reported by chronic headache sufferers. Elite runners, on the other
hand, paid especially close attention to bodily sensations arising in
their feet, calves, and chest. They repeatedly reminded themselves to
relax and "stay loose" during the run.

Psychobiological aspects of migraine are often mistaken by sufferers as being synonymous with a psychological explanation of their condition, leading to the fear that the disorder will be minimized or blamed on them. This situation will change only with improved understanding of the meaning and nature of the psychobiological determinants of headache disorders.

What Is the Psychobiological Significance of a Migraine Headache?

What is the body trying to tell the individual who has recurring headaches for no apparent reason? A reasonable hypothesis is that headache is the expression of a bodily need for sleep or, in holistic terms, the psychobiological need for self-soothing. Migraine episodes are often preceded by yawning and fatigue, suggesting the involvement of hypothalamic sleep mechanisms. These symptoms are often present upon awakening and may be accompanied by neck tightness, nausea, and feverlike sensations. The headache-alleviating power of sleep has been known for a long time. In 1863, John Hilton published a classic text titled *Rest and Pain,* with the theme that rest for an injured tissue is essential to its recovery (Walls & Philipp, 1953). It is common knowledge that sleep is the most effective natural means for alleviating acute headache episodes. If sleep is not possible, then behavioral withdrawal from work, family, and noise is the next best step.

It is surprising how few chronic migraine and tension headache sufferers benefit from a night's sleep or daytime rest. Some of these individuals complain that the pain is worse after sleep or rest. Clearly, sleep of any kind will not do. Headache sufferers generally do not sleep well and many report the beginnings of headache upon awakening. The sleep of these individuals has been characterized as nonrestorative rather than restorative in nature. A similar nonrestorative sleep pattern is reported to characterize the musculoskeletal symptoms that fibromyalgia sufferers experience upon awakening (Moldofksy, 1989). Described as a miserable flulike feeling, the condition is characterized by headache, generalized muscle aching, tiredness, nervousness, and irritability. Research is required to determine the characteristics of sleep that are associated with good and poor headache relief. For example, analgesics and other medications taken for headache and sleep could be a factor in the symptoms on waking, with increased headache being generated as the individual withdraws from the medicine. Also of concern is the psychological state of headache sufferers prior to and during sleep. Clinical evidence suggests the presence of considerable anxiety, worry, and depression in these individuals. Headache sufferers seldom connect their condition with a need for better sleep or the need to pay attention to bodily events associated with beginning headache.

In a graduate class discussion of the potential power of somatic awareness for preventing migraine, I remarked that most migraine sufferers have difficulty maintaining the level of awareness required to minimize the occurrence of headache attacks. Migraine sufferers, like everyone else, are too often caught up in the demands of daily living to make the necessary changes within themselves to prevent future attacks. The students seemed surprised that migraineurs would not readily make use of awareness of bodily sensations, especially if this awareness led to a reduction in the frequency and severity of painful and sickening headache attacks. At the end of class, I gave one of the students, who happened to suffer from migraine, a relaxation tape for home practice of somatic awareness. During the next class, I asked the student about her experiences with the tape. She replied in an apologetic fashion that the tape was still sitting, unheard, on the coffee table in her home. She had been too busy that week but "promised" to get to it—as soon as she could find some time.

This student's situation is representative of what is commonly seen with patients who are asked to take steps to care for themselves. They feel that they do not have the time to make the necessary changes. Learning to make psychobiological changes within oneself can paradoxically be the simplest and most difficult of adjustments an individual will ever make. Once the decision is made to utilize bodily information, however, the experiential state becomes easier to initiate and to maintain throughout the waking and sleeping states. Somatic awareness, following some initial practice, can quickly become an automatic component of an individual's conscious experience.

REDUCING THE PAIN OF CHILDBIRTH

The pain experienced during childbirth labor has been described as one of the most intense of all clinical pain conditions, exceeded only by nerve pain and amputation (Melzack, 1984). Somatic awareness has the potential not only to reduce the pain of childbirth but also to make the process more efficient (i.e., shorter), safer, and less stressful on mother and newborn

Recent childbirth studies indicate that *attention toward* rather than *avoidance* of physical sensations is a necessary first step to reducing the pain of childbirth. The research of Leventhal and colleagues (Leventhal, Leventhal, Shacham, & Easterling, 1989) initiated this new understanding. In their study, women about to experience childbirth labor pain were assigned to sensory monitoring or sensory distraction groups to see which group experienced less pain. The sensory monitoring group was provided the following instructions:

> I want you to pay close attention to specific aspects of your contractions. You can see how often they come, but more importantly, you should pay close attention to how they feel ... to where you feel them. ... Do this with each of your contractions. ... These sensations are not necessarily the same as pain, so be sure to focus on them. Paying attention to your contractions shouldn't interfere with relaxing and breathing but should help you to regulate and guide these behaviors. (p. 367)

Women assigned to the monitoring group reported less pain than women assigned to the distraction group. Leventhal et al. hypothesized that body stimuli are processed for both sensory informational features and emotional or threatening value. Sensory monitoring may intercept the formation of higher order interpretations and result in a "detached" self-view, draining the higher order meaning out of somatic experience. Sensory monitoring results in a relatively neutral perception of the situation, and thereby defuses the cost of a negative and emotional interpretation of it. Sensory monitoring is able, under appropriate instruction, to alter the physiological and subjective reactions associated with the emotional processing arm of the pain system (Leventhal, 1993).

Somatic awareness may be used to improve both the experience and the efficacy of childbirth. The labor experience can be painful and frightening, and there is some evidence that general distress is associated with less efficient or longer labors. Moreover, there is evidence that high levels of pain and distress during early, or latent, labor interferes with the natural labor process. Latent labor is characterized by cervical dilatation of 3 centimeters or less and contractions that are less frequent and regular than those in active labor. The active phase of labor, which is usually defined by dilatation between 3 and 10 centimeters, averages between 3 and 4 hours in length. Descriptive studies have reported that the latent phase of labor lasts 9–10 hours in normal nulliparous women (Wuitchik, Bakal, & Lipshitz, 1989). But women show enormous variability in the length of this phase, ranging from less than 1 hour to close to 30 hours.

Women's pain levels during latent labor are generally not considered clinically significant for understanding the total childbirth experience; pain reported during active labor is considered clinically more important. There is some evidence, however, that pain levels during latent labor correlate with the length of latent labor. Women reporting *excruciating* pain during this phase go on to have a mean latent labor length of 14.4 hours while women who reported pain as *discomforting* had a mean latent labor length of 6.5 hours (Wuitchik et al., 1989).

One hypothesis in need of investigation is whether increased somatic awareness during early labor might not only lessen the level of pain experienced but also facilitate the labor process. Women are often taught or encouraged to distract from sensory/bodily processes (e.g., focus on nonbody images, external points, patterned paced breathing). These attempts at distraction and active control might actually serve to separate the mother from the physiological sensations (and processes) of labor itself. There is also a risk that dissociative techniques, while effective in the short run, will fail as the demands of labor increase, resulting in increased fear, distress, and pain. In a pilot investigation, we examined whether women's attentional focus during labor might be predictive of length of latent labor (Hesson, Hill, & Bakal, 1997). Attentional focus was assessed by asking women to describe their thoughts between contractions. The thoughts were then examined for *associative* (attention to body information and use of that information to facilitate relaxation and/or manage contractions) or *dissociative* (avoidance or distraction from body sensations) content.

Examples of the two different cognitive styles are presented in Table 1.1. Women who employed associative strategies paid close attention to their breathing, as well as to sensations of tension in various body parts. They then used this information to regulate their breathing

TABLE 1.1. Examples of Associative and Dissociative Coping Styles Reported during Contractions

Associative strategies

"I am thinking about breathing slowly and relaxing my muscles—trying to keep the same steady breathing."

"Making sure I get lots of oxygen and relaxing . . . concentrating on Andy's fingers massaging my back . . . going on to the next one."

"Concentrating on breathing—telling self I have to breathe in this fashion until pain subsides downwards."

Dissociative strategies

"I'm trying the breathing, but when the pain is excruciating, I do anything to focus my mind away."

"I'm thinking about how painful it is and when will it be over—I did concentrate on breathing, but I found that distraction feels better."

"Focusing on Dave's face and the numbers . . . what the next number is because we are counting."

Note. Adapted from Hesson, Hill, and Bakal (1997). Copyright 1997 by the American College of Nurse–Midwives. Adapted by permission of Elsevier Science.

and facilitate relaxation. Women employing dissociative strategies, on the other hand, tended to focus on events external to themselves, such as their spouse's behavior. The most frequently reported cognition of the dissociative group had to do with how much longer the labor was going to last.

The two groups of women differed in terms of their respiration rate during latent labor. The women in the associative group had an average respiration rate of 14.9 cycles per minute between contractions and 12.8 cycles per minute during contractions. The women in the dissociative group had an average respiration rate of 20.5 cycles per minute between contractions and 23.7 cycles per minute during contractions. The two groups also differed in their total labor lengths. Although the difference was nonsignificant, the associative group's labor length was shorter on average by 2 hours than the dissociative group's labor length.

WELLNESS WITHIN THE SKIN

We need to continue searching for ways of teaching the public to appreciate the health-promoting and healing potential of somatic awareness. We have been grossly unimaginative in our ways of thinking and theorizing about the body. Patients in particular need to understand that it is all right for them to listen to their bodies and to take care of themselves. There is no single step for achieving body awareness: it can come through an overall change of personality or through limited adjustments in dealing with bodily symptoms. In all cases there needs to be greater utilization of bodily information as a legitimate dimension of health promotion.

I believe that somatic awareness is a universal health promotion process within the skin that can be readily identified by all individuals. Somatic awareness, however, is not the mental equivalent of the pharmacological "magic bullet" or the cure-all for every illness condition. Somatic awareness is best viewed as an experiential guide in helping the individual maximize his or her inner resources in the prevention of and recovery from illness. There is no magic dietary formula, mental phrase, prayer, breathing pattern, or body movement that guarantees healing across individuals. Each person must find his or her own path. Health professionals need to be active collaborators in this discovery process.

Some psychophysiological disorders, for example, migraine headache and asthma, are readily linked to bodily sensations and therefore are more readily managed through somatic awareness directed toward the underlying pathophysiology (e.g., muscle tightness, restricted breathing). Other illnesses, for example, hypertension and heart disease, have less readily identifiable sensory correlates of pathophysiological mechanisms. With these conditions, it is necessary to identify bodily sensations that are indirectly or secondarily related to underlying disease processes. In the case of heart disease, for example, the individual may need to work with chest sensations that are indirectly related to angina. By learning how to use stress management techniques and not to attribute the arousal sensations of living (e.g., exercise, sexual activity) as indicative of heart failure, individuals may be able to limit or even reverse coronary artherosclerosis. Finally, there are a large number of chronic and life-threatening diseases associated with the immune system that seem to have little or no connection to bodily sensations. We are not normally aware of the status of our immune system. In these instances, somatic awareness needs to be conceptualized in broad nonspecific terms and its health benefits experienced more in terms of general well-being rather than in terms of localized sensations.

We know that people can readily identify illness-related bodily sensations that they associate with feelings of chronic fatigue, depression, "being stressed out," and "being uptight." It stands to reason that they can learn to experience the absence or opposite of such feelings. The existence of a general state of psychobiological wellness, experienced through somatic awareness, although not as yet demonstrable through scientific methodology, is consistent with clinical reports and writings. Countless clinical publications attest to the therapeutic value of similar soothing strategies based on imagery, belief, and relaxation in the treatment of a wide range of symptoms, disorders, and diseases. The fact that the same or similar interventions have at least some success with physical conditions of widely different biological origins points to a powerful communality in the treatment of many medical conditions.

There are many other variables both outside and within a person that deflect attention from the use of inner body experience to attain health. These include external stress, internal anxiety and fear surrounding the meaning of bodily information, and widespread differences in personal coping styles. However, it remains possible to promote somatic awareness as a health-enhancing strategy across all individuals, regardless of their circumstances. Whether dealing with interpersonal and situational stress, emotional conditions, chronic pain disorders, immune system disorders, or life-threatening disease, somatic awareness constitutes an important holistic dimension that can be used to guide therapeutic efforts designed to attain symptom management and improve health. In giving centrality to body sensations, I am not minimizing the importance of a person's thoughts, feelings, and behaviors, or of the social context in which these actions take place. To the contrary, I am emphasizing somatic awareness as a way of identifying the psychobiological processes that mediate between psychosocial factors and illness and maximize the individual's intrinsic healing systems.

Some experts believe that approaches such as mine that emphasize wellness within the skin place too much pressure on the individual in the search for health. Antonovsky (1994) challenged the wisdom of the individual approach on the grounds that it results in insufficient attention being given to the larger social system in which the mind–body relationship operates. Society, according to Antonovsky, is a more appropriate system level to influence because changes at the societal level can eventually make their way to each individual's inner conscious life in a more egalitarian fashion. Antonovsky argues that it is not fair to expect the disadvantaged, the marginalized, the victimized, the sick, and the homeless to "take care of themselves" through somatic awareness or any other individual means. Others have echoed a similar concern that "mind over matter courses" cannot always expect individuals to "perceive away" a reality that is unacceptable. It is unreasonable, they insist, to mouth platitudes about self-help and wellness to people who are overwhelmed by unsolvable societal and/or medical problems.

Antonovsky (1994) described the pressure of searching for health within ourselves as a "new version of Freudianism"—a looking within the skin that prevents people from understanding the social pressures and events beyond their control that cause people to behave in a pathogenic fashion. He believes that in its most extreme form the emphasis on seeking health within is immoral, especially when consideration is given to the socially disadvantaged. He provides an example from the Midtown Manhattan Study, which found over a 20-year period an intergenerational improvement in mental health not because of the increased use of mind control or stress management courses but because of the societal improvement in women's status and their share of resources. Changes in social class, gender roles, and minority status made the difference.

Another relevant example for women's health is the repeated demonstration of a relationship between physical and psychological abuse and health status. Several studies have found a relationship between abuse history in women and physical health disorders, pain disorders, and psychiatric illness (Leserman et al., 1996). Less tangible forms of psychological abuse might be operating to explain the high incidence of a number of other illnesses in women. Women continue to bear the burden of caring for their children, working, and finally often having to care for sick and dying spouses and family members. Women still lack sufficient time to care for themselves.

At a philosophical level, I have considerable empathy for the Antonovsky argument. Our society places too much emphasis on individuality and survival, without sufficient regard for social, economic, and environmental inequalities across people. Advocating somatic awareness in health does not mean that the larger social system is unimportant and health is exclusively the property of the individual. We know, for example, that psychosocial variables involving community, family, work, and peers make a very significant difference in terms of health and illness. Taylor, Repetti, and Seeman (1997), following their review of the environmental literature, concluded that environments that provide safety, opportunities for social integration, and the ability to predict and/or control are most likely to contribute to health. People cannot be expected to assume responsibility for factors outside their own control. Moreover, people should not blame themselves when they are afflicted with an illness, and they certainly should not experience guilt in feeling that they cannot cure themselves.

Although my discussion has focused on factors within the individual, I conceptualize somatic awareness as a dimension of bodily health that depends on both psychosocial factors outside the skin and psychobiological factors within the skin. I view the maintenance of health as a complex balancing act involving many factors controlled by the mind and the body. Somatic awareness is an emergent property of mind–body function that is central to the individual's effort to balance these factors in an effort to maintain health and well-being. Somatic awareness is not a new concept: it was recognized by early Greek philosophers. It is also in the background of current developments in holistic health. Today, no matter which medical symptom or chronic disease is being discussed, there is a greater recognition that psychological stress is involved and that similar stress-management techniques can be used to treat the condition under discussion. Surely, there must be common psychobiological processes at work.

Somatic awareness is one of the most natural aspects of consciousness. Although language limitations, vague physiological origins, fear of the body, dualistic beliefs, disease attributions, and life's "external" demands can interfere, bodily awareness and self-soothing remain fundamental processes of conscious life. The healing potential of the somatic awareness heuristic is immense. We will see in the following chapters that somatic awareness has significant implications for (1) understanding common medical symptoms, (2) developing new models of drug action, (3) explaining placebo power, (4) preventing and maximizing recovery from immune system diseases, and (5) providing health professionals with a holistic framework for patient care.

CHAPTER 2

Somatization

THE NATURE OF SOMATIZATION

A middle aged man presents to emergency clinic with heart palpitations and chest pain, upon which electrocardiographic (ECG) investigation prove to have no cardiac cause.

A young woman presents with symptoms of dizziness and nausea upon awakening. The failure to resolve her symptoms has led to fears of an undiagnosed medical disease.

An elderly patient while watching TV in hospital suddenly begins to sweat, and while making his way back to his room falls in the corridor. No physical cause of the episode is found.

A widowed 67-year-old woman with liver cancer, living alone, begins to experience, in the early hours of the morning, chest and abdominal pain, and diarrhea. Although the cancer is untreatable, her oncologist believes the present symptoms are not the result of the cancer. She fears that the bodily symptoms are evidence of the cancer eating from within.

These clinical vignettes serve to illustrate the diverse nature of symptom presentations associated with somatization. Somatization, described throughout the history of medicine, generally refers to symptoms that occur in the absence of a physical cause. There are actually a very large number of troublesome physiological symptoms that occur in the absence of an identifiable medical cause. Because of the lack of a medical cause, the presence of somatization symptoms creates considerable frustration and confusion in health professionals who are trying to understand the symptoms and the patients who are experiencing the symptoms. In many respects, somatization is an example of somatic awareness gone awry. My goal in this chapter is to provide a framework for understanding and managing patients who present with somatization symptoms. The individual's body is reacting at some level to situational and/or emotional stress, but the reaction is taking place outside of conscious awareness. The body is only "noticed" once the reactions reach symptomatic or illness level, as in the case of dizziness, abdominal pain, and the like. Furthermore, the individual at this point does not understand the symptom and becomes frightened about its presence. There is no understanding that bodily attention might be utilized to alleviate or prevent the symptom.

We lack a satisfactory model for explaining and managing physical symptoms in the absence of physical cause. Patients with such symptoms have been variously described as "hypochondriacal," "neurotic," "hysterical," or "functional"—the common theme being that the symptoms serve some unconscious symbolic function for the person, such as masking depression or hostility or, through the sick role, attracting attention and/or providing the means to manipulate others.

Wilhelm Stekel coined the term "somatization" in 1911 and defined it as "the process by which neurotic conflicts may present themselves as a physical disorder" (van der Feltz-Cornelis & van Dyck, 1997). Stekel regarded somatization as identical to what Freud called "conversion." Somatization is currently defined as a general tendency to experience and communicate emotional distress in terms of somatic discomfort (Piccinelli & Simon, 1997). The psychobiological processes involved in somatization are generally unconscious rather than conscious.

Patient presentations of somatic symptoms associated with dizziness, fainting, pain, and shortness of breath are very common occurrences. Kroenke (1992), an internal medicine specialist, remarked that "symptoms are among the leading reasons patients visit doctors, yet are among the last things a doctor wants to see." This tongue-in-cheek statement conveys the frustration physicians and patients alike feel in trying to understand and manage somatic symptoms that occur in the absence of an identifiable physical cause. Patients with symptoms that have no basis in identifiable pathophysiology may constitute over half of all patients who visit primary care physicians. The incidence may even be higher, for many patients do not mention all their symptoms when they present to clinics for diagnostic tests, examinations, and procedures. Symptoms without medical cause also occur with great frequency in the general population. Community data show a lifetime prevalence of close to 25% for chest pain, back pain, dizziness, headache, and abdominal pain. The incidence of these symptoms is much higher in the clinic, with at least 80% of patients surveyed admitting to at least one somatic symptom involving dyspnea (labored breathing), chest pain, abdominal pain, headache, dizziness, back pain, or fatigue (Kroenke, 1992).

Somatization is recognized as a worldwide phenomenon (Kirmayer, 1984). Somatic symptoms are more common than emotional complaints as a way of presenting psychological stress. In some cultures, somatic symptoms seem to be the only means by which a person can express psychological distress because these cultures lack adequate language to describe all emotional states (Janca, Isac, Bennett, & Tacchini, 1995). Some of the more common somatization symptoms that occur across cultures involve sleep disturbance, tension headaches, back pain, and indigestion. It is also very common for individuals across cultures to refuse psychological explanations for these symptoms (Janca et al., 1995).

Diagnostic testing for somatic symptoms, although necessary, seldom leads to a physical cause and medical treatment seldom results in satisfactory resolution of the symptom. Kroenke and Mangelsdorff (1989) reviewed the incidence data of 1,000 patients who presented to an internal medicine clinic with at least 1 of 14 somatic symptoms. The incidence data ranged from 1.2% to 9.6% per symptom. A physical or organic cause was detected infrequently for the most common symptoms. In addition, it was also shown through a follow-up study that the percentage of improvement or satisfaction with treatment was generally less than 50%. Somatic symptoms are seldom resolved in medical settings and many patients become frustrated with their health care professionals. Professionals' efforts to explain these symptoms as manifestations of psychological stress or anxiety, unconscious conflicts, family dysfunction, or faulty thinking styles causes patients to feel that their condition has been misunderstood. They resent the inference that their bodily symptoms have no "real" basis and exist only in their head. The need for a better understanding of somatic experiences is evident from the familiar patient plea "If nothing physical is wrong, then what is wrong? I have no reason to be anxious and I don't think I am depressed."

Many authors have pointed to the presentation of somatic symptoms as evidence of depression or what is called "masked depression." For example, it has been repeatedly suggested that Chinese patients tend to express depression in somatic terms, interpreting somatic concomitants of depression such as dry mouth, musculoskeletal pain, fatigue, impaired concentration, headache, and dizziness as signs of nervous weakness while minimizing or denying their emotional concerns. This failure to report psychological symptoms has been attributed to the social and moral stigma attached to emotional complaints in Chinese culture. There are anecdotal reports of high rates of somatization in other Asian cultures. For example, somatic symptoms involving pressure on the head, headache, shoulder pain, feelings of coldness, fatigue, and dizziness are characteristic of Japanese women. Such symptoms are most often interpreted as indicative of depression. In India, the sensation of bodily heat or burning is a common bodily symptom. In Iran, patients report a sensation of "a strong hard hand squeezing their hearts." Saudi women frequently complain of fatigue and head, neck, and back pain, symptoms that have been attributed to their limited opportunity for expression of emotional distress.

It is unknown whether some cultures are more prone to somatization than others. In North America, close to 80% of college students report some degree of at least one of a number of common medical symptoms (headache, upset stomach, sore muscles, nasal congestion, flushed face, dizziness, sweaty hands, shortness of breath, watering eyes, ringing in ears) when sampled during classroom lectures. Bodily symptoms are a normal experience even for individuals in good health. The fact that the majority of these students do not seek treatment for their symptoms suggests that we are dealing with complex processes in differentiating those who seek/need medical attention and those who do not.

Neurasthenia was a frequent somatization disorder diagnosis in the late 1800s. It was considered a physical disorder caused by overwork, bereavement, family difficulties, and other debilitating physical illnesses that depleted "nervous force" and resulted in a variety of physical illnesses including abdominal pain, heartburn, nausea and vomiting, insomnia, and paresthesias. Classical neurasthenia is likely still very much with us in the form of chronic fatigue, exhaustion and "burnout." The symptoms of neurasthenia include bodily weakness, fatigue, tiredness, headaches, dizziness, and a number of gastrointestinal and other complaints. Neurasthenia remains a very common diagnosis in China, where it is called "shenjing shuairuo," which means neurological weakness. Mexican Americans and Puerto Ricans describe similar symptoms as occurrences of *nervios,* or nervousness (Matsumi & Draguns, 1996).

A purely psychological defense perspective would see neurasthenia as "a face-saving organic diagnosis for experiences of exhaustion, demoralization or depression in cultures that equate energy with prestige" (Kirmayer, 1984, p. 175). Although such a definition is too narrow to capture the full range of psychobiological processes contributing to neurasthenia or somatization, the emphasis on psychological factors illustrates the reality that somatic discomfort, social conflict, and existential neurosis tend to co-occur in the same individual. Somatization thus involves a very complex interplay between physiological mechanisms associated with both somatic and emotional symptoms, cognitive attributional processes, and social processes that encourage or sanction particular styles of expressing distress. This description of the systemic nature of somatization is similar to the description of somatic awareness provided in the opening chapter. It is not easy to keep the meaning of the two terms separate. However, in contrast to somatization, somatic awareness is a positive volitional process, with the purpose of alleviating symptom presence and restoring feelings of well-being.

Psychiatry has always, by nature of the discipline, viewed the body in negative or symptomatic terms. Psychiatry has a diagnostic category called "somatization disorder" that constitutes a more current description of clinical conditions associated with classical hypochondriasis and hysteria. Assigning a diagnosis of somatization disorder is a complex and arbitrary process. It requires that the patient present with a symptom complex characterized by a combination of symptoms that includes pain related to at least four different sites (e.g., head, abdomen, back, chest, rectum), two gastrointestinal symptoms (e.g., nausea, bloating), one sexual/reproductive symptom (e.g., irregular menses, premature ejaculation), and one "pseudoneurological" symptom (e.g., impaired balance, localized weakness). None of these symptoms can have a medical cause or be due to substance abuse, and none must intentionally feigned or produced (American Psychiatric Association, 1994). Not surprisingly, few individuals meet this strict definition. Indeed, most people who present with more limited symptoms to their general practitioner do not show evidence of having a psychiatric somatization disorder.

There are two major psychiatric models of somatization, one based on classical ideas of conversion and defense and the other based on more recent notions of cognitive misattribution. The defense model views the somatic symptom as occurring in place of personal or social problems, while the misattribution model emphasizes the negative attributions or cognitions that individuals make toward their physical symptoms (Simon, 1991). Regardless of theoretical orientation, somatization is often inferred when the clinician suspects that the source of the problem lies in emotional distress or interpersonal conflicts, despite the patient's pointing to a body part in response to the question, "Where does it hurt?" With the elderly, it is a common practice to assume that undiagnosed somatic complaints are indicative of depression. In both viewpoints, the afflicted individual is considered to have no awareness of the nature of the psychobiological processes contributing to the symptom's development and maintenance.

The idea that the occurrence of a somatic symptom reflects a form of psychological defense constitutes the traditional approach to somatization phenomena (Simon, 1991). Within this model, "out of mind" does not mean "out of body." The opposite is true in that bodily symptoms allow the person to express mental distress without having to acknowledge underlying depression or anxiety. For example, patients who present with intractable pain, have been described as suffering from a number of psychological conflicts of which they are unaware. The pain is seen as a form of *masked* depression, hostility, guilt, resentment, or the like. According to Engel (1959), their developmental experiences cause some individuals to use pain unconsciously to resolve conflicts. These conflicts might involve aggression, guilt, or fear of threatened loss of a relationship. Although the majority of accumulated data fails to find much evidence in support of the notion that unconscious emotional conflicts give rise to pain, early traumatic experiences may influence the way an individual experiences pain and suffering, should a pain disorder develop. It is remarkable how many chronic pain patients who experience considerable suffering in association with their chronic pain have also experienced early childhood trauma and/or lifelong psychological abuse. Clinicians should always investigate the possibility of early and lifelong abuse with chronic pain patients. In women in particular there is evidence that a history of sexual and/or physical abuse are associated with pronounced chronic pain (Linton, 1997).

At the same time, trying to view a patient's physical symptom as having a specific psychological cause, such as depression, is too narrow an approach. In spite of the difficulties surrounding efforts to link specific emotions, personalities, and life experiences to specific bodily symptoms, clinicians working with somatic awareness must always remain open to a whole range of past and present psychobiological determinants of symptoms. Symptoms such as pain, fatigue, nausea, insomnia, and irritable bowel, although linked to a patient's thoughts and feelings, seldom develop in response to a specific psychological difficulty. It is true that patients who present with somatic symptoms often acknowledge difficulties with depression, anxiety, anger, and irritability, but these emotional states are not necessarily *the reason* for the physical symptom. It is best to view the link between emotionality and symptom development indirectly through a form of collateral psychobiological discharge. Physiologists use the term "collateral" to describe pathways that contribute to nonspecific activation regions such as the somatosensory cortex and the noradrenergic pathways. Any emotional state is thus capable of contributing to symptom onset in the vulnerable individual. In the same vein, self-regulation of the symptom via somatic awareness of these psychobiological pathways becomes a distinct possibility.

Amplification of Distress

The view toward nonspecific distress rather than specific psychological conflicts in the study of somatization is evident in the *amplification of distress* model of somatization (Simon, 1991). Within this model it is assumed that somatic and subjective distress co-occur rather than substitute for one another. This model assumes that patients who present with somatic complaints also present with high levels of subjective complaints. This model is the opposite of the traditional unconscious defense model which assumes that the presentation of physical symptoms is a substitute for the presentation of psychological symptoms. In the amplification model, psychological distress is experienced fully in consciousness. As discussed later, this model has its flaws but it also offers some insights into the interaction of psychological and physical complaints in some individuals.

Support for the positive relationship between expressions of psychological and physical symptoms comes from community survey studies. Simon and Von Korff (1991) used data from the National Institute of Mental Health Epidemiologic Catchment Area Study to examine the relationship between somatization and the report of psychiatric symptoms in a multisite community survey. A structured clinical interview was used to assess the presence of psychiatric diagnoses. Panic disorder, obsessive compulsive disorder, and phobia were diagnosed from the anxiety disorders included in the diagnostic system. Symptoms from panic and phobia sections were combined to produce a single anxiety symptom count. When current emotional problems and psychiatric symptoms were combined, nearly 75% of the high somatizing group showed current psychological distress. Respondents reporting the greatest number of somatic symptoms also had the highest risk for panic disorder. Only a small number of respondents with high levels of somatization failed to report anxiety or depressive symptoms. Research of this nature suggests that anxiety and panic are important—if not *the* most important—determinants of somatization

Piccinelli and Simon (1997) examined psychological and somatic symptom data obtained from 14 countries around the world as part of the World Health Organization Collaborative Project on Psychological Problems in General Health Care. Data on levels of emotional distress and somatic symptoms were obtained from 5,190 subjects. Emotional distress was assessed with a standardized questionnaire that contained anxiety and depression subscales. The sum of the items from the two scales was used as an index of emotional distress. A structured clinical interview was used to assess for the presence of 22 somatic symptoms. The symptoms reflected four symptom groups: gastrointestinal, neurological, musculoskeletal, and autonomic. Overall emotional distress and somatic symptom scores correlated positively across all centers. Females tended to report more somatic symptoms than males at each level of emotional distress. The study provided additional support for the notion that emotional and somatic symptoms tend to occur together.

Costa and McCrae (1987) postulated that the distress–somatization covariation observed in normal and patient samples is due to neuroticism. They defined "neuroticism" as a chronic condition of irritability and distress-proneness that operates independently of signs of real physical illness. That is, neuroticism or negative affectivity is associated with the verbal report of both psychological and physical problems but is not necessarily associated with the presence of more physical disease. The anxious individual, in their words, has a perceptual bias and "seeks out and amplifies bodily sensations." In a similar fashion, Barsky (1992) hypothesized that the presentation of benign physical symptoms such as palpitation and chest pain is associated with somatosensory amplification and misattribution. Some individuals are prone to exaggerate or amplify sensations that would otherwise be experienced as benign and nonthreatening by the nonanxious individual. "Bodily amplification" is defined as the tendency to experience benign bodily sensations as noxious and intense and encompasses three components: (1) bodily hypervigilance that involves heightened self-scrutiny; (2) a tendency to select out and focus on certain relatively mild or infrequent sensations; and (3) a tendency to experience bodily sensation as abnormal and symptomatic of disease.

Barsky's (1992) notion of amplification is similar to the formulations of other theorists who invoke cognitive concepts like perceptual bias and misattribution to explain symptom development in the absence of disease. Barsky described how such beliefs might operate in the general population to influence decisions to seek medical attention:

> Amplification might also be salient in the pathogenesis of several ambiguous conditions that are of unclear clinical status and significance, such as irritable bowel syndrome, fibromyalgia, hypoglycemia, and chronic fatigue syndrome. These conditions are confusing because there are apparently many people in the community with the same complaints who have never sought medical attention for them. It is possible that it is the

perceived intensity of their symptoms (e.g., abdominal cramps, lighthead-edness, musculoskeletal pain, fatigue) that distinguishes those who go to doctors from those who do not. Perhaps it is the amplification of these ubiquitous complaints by a few hypersensitive individuals that gives the symptoms clinical significance. It has been suggested, for example, that irritable bowel syndrome patients amplify mild and benign gut dysfunction and that they are hypersensitive to distention of the gut or to smooth muscle contraction in the bowel wall. (p. 32)

Beliefs do make a significant difference in determining how individuals deal with symptoms. However, in working with cognitive concepts like amplification and misattribution, we need to be careful not to assume that the bodily sensations reported by patients have no physiological underpinnings. Cognitive concepts are important, but they can foster a form of dualism by implying that a physiological substrate to the symptom experience may not exist. Barsky, for example, often refers to the underlying physiology as being *benign* or *normal,* which implies that nothing significant is taking place at the physiological level. Within his framework, symptom presentation depends not on physiological change, but instead on how the patient interprets and reacts to normal physiological events. It cannot be assumed, however, that because a patient's descriptive phenomenological experiences with body symptoms are often difficult to describe and are subject to misinterpretation or amplification, the physiological origins of these experiences are unimportant. It is possible that the reverse is true: the more difficult it is for the patient to describe the experience, the more likely it is that something significant at a physiological level is taking place. Individuals who develop frightening thoughts surrounding their internal bodily sensations often do so because the physiological processes contributing to these sensations are experienced as being outside of their control and consequently dangerous. We will see that there is usually much more taking place physiologically than what one would observe as a "normal" bodily response.

A more serious limitation of the amplification model is the fact that not all individuals with somatization symptoms engage in thinking characterized by amplification of their symptoms. It may be the case that the majority of individuals do not amplify during presentation or discussion of their somatic symptoms. Indeed, a significant percentage of the population with unexplained somatic symptoms attempts to ignore or minimize rather than to amplify the emotional significance of their symptoms. That is, many individuals with somatic symptoms express little or no exaggeration or amplification of their physical symptom. If anything, they deny or avoid thinking about its existence.

Hypnotizability and Threat Perception

Wickramasekera (1995) attempted to integrate the different forms that somatization may take. His model accounts for overrecognition and underrecognition of psychological contributions to somatic symptoms through the dimensions of hypnotic susceptibility and negative affectivity. Wickramasekera believes that extreme positions on the hypnotic susceptibility continuum are indicative of individuals who are at risk for somatization. He postulates that individuals who are highly hypnotizable have a tendency to amplify somatic sensations, and individuals who are low in terms of hypnotizability have a tendency to deny subjective distress and to minimize somatic sensations. The risk for somatization is greatest in highly hypnotizable individuals who also exhibit negative affectivity, that is, the tendency to chronically experience negative emotions such as anxiety, fear, anger or depression, even when there is no clear experiential trigger for such feelings. Hypnotic susceptibility is associated with a thinking style characterized by a sense of involuntariness or perceived lack of control when under threat. This thinking style puts such individuals at risk for involuntary changes in perception, memory, and mood that can amplify the perception of fear and pain. This amplification of fear and pain can trigger the hypothalamic-pituitary-adrenal axis and alter immune function and, when confronted with threat may spontaneously activate the hypnotic mode of information processing and experience.

Wickramasekera's model is less developed for individuals who are low in hypnotic susceptibility. However, he follows traditional thinking in postulating that these are individuals who are nonexpressive with respect to psychological distress but who may be quite reactive physiologically in the face of threat:

> I hypothesize that lows are hyposensitive consciously or verbally, but not implicitly or sympathetically, to relevant threats. Yet, they repress or deny psychological causation. They prefer mechanical, surgical, or chemical solutions to their problems. Threat perception in lows may be absent from verbal report or consciousness but present in measures of sympathetic activation or motor behavior. (p. 16)

To test his model, Wickramasekera (1995) identified a sample of medical somatizers, that is, patients who had previously been medically investigated. These patients suffered from a broad spectrum of somatic and psychological symptom complaints, including headaches, fainting (negative CT scans), asthma, chronic pain, insomnia, vomiting, angina (negative cardiac catheterization), anxiety, depression, and panic. Their symptoms had not responded to conventional medical therapies.

Hypnotic ability was assessed using the Harvard Group Scale of Hypnotic Susceptibility (Hilgard & Hilgard, 1975) and compared to the hypnotic susceptibility scores of a matched community sample of individuals who attended a conference on stress management. The hypnotic susceptibility scores for the community sample followed a normal distribution, with the majority of individuals obtaining moderate hypnotic susceptibility scores. The somatizers, on the other hand, were more likely than the controls to occupy positions of low or high hypnotic susceptibility. Somatizers in the low and high hypnotic susceptibility groups manifested a higher percentage of somatic than psychological symptoms than somatizers in the moderate hypnotic susceptibility group. Patients in the low and high susceptibility groups exhibited higher percentages of somatic symptoms than psychological symptoms (96% vs. 4% for lows; 76% vs. 24% for highs).

Wickramasekera (1995) believes that patients with high hypnotic susceptibility scores are more responsive than patients low in hypnotic susceptibility to therapies designed to utilize somatic awareness. He argues that they are better able than low hypnotic susceptibility patients to redirect their "hypnotic talent" from illness to health. With guidance, they became adept at using cognitive reappraisal and relaxation skills to access and defuse unconscious perceptions of current threat and memories of past threat: "They learn that it is not enough to put out the 'fire' (symptoms) with hypnotic or biofeedback skills, but they must also learn to find the 'matches' (identify and define unconscious threats) to avoid new symptoms, because out of mind is not out of body" (p. 21).

The determinants of hypnotic talent and its relationship to somatic awareness are not clear. It does appear, however, that Wickramasekera is speaking of an individual difference parameter that directly influences the perception of bodily sensations. Low hypnotic susceptibility patients, he maintains, are much more difficult to treat with any form of psychological intervention, including somatic awareness training. In the extreme form, individuals who present with physical symptoms in the complete absence of psychological complaints are referred to as manifesting *alexithymia*.

ALEXITHYMIA AND SOMATIC AWARENESS

"Alexithymia" is a term first coined by Sifneos (1973, 1996) to refer to a disturbance in psychobiological functioning characterized by difficulties in the capacity to experience and verbalize affect. The word *alexithymia* is derived from the Greek *a* for lack, *lexis* for word, and *thymos* for feeling. Absence of body awareness, called "alexisomia," may also characterize the condition. The difficulty goes beyond mere nonexpressiveness as these individuals have difficulty identifying and describing their own feelings:

> It became apparent that alexithymic individuals had a major deficit in both their capacity to experience, differentiate, and describe feelings, and their ability to create fantasy. As a consequence of those deficits, stressful arousal was directly transformed into somatic dysfunction without the intervening psychological elaboration characteristic of neurotic symptom formation. Metaphorically speaking, alexithymic persons had no psychodynamic upper story. (Nemiah, 1996, p. 217)

A number of studies indicate that alexithymia is related to physical symptoms and subjective reports of poor health. For example, alexithymia has been found to be predictive of greater risk of all-cause death in a community sample of men in Finland (Kauhanen, Kaplan, Cohen, Julkunen, & Salonen, 1996). Kauhanen et al. are not able to explain why difficulties in dealing with emotions increase mortality, but they believe the link is independent of behavioral (e.g., smoking, physical activity), biological (e.g., high-density lipoprotein, low-density lipoprotein, hypertension), and psychosocial (e.g., marital status, depression) risk factors. Lumley, Stettner, and Wehmer (1996) suggested four pathways that may account for the relationship between alexithymia and physical illness. They separate physical illness into *organic disease* characterized by tissue pathology and *illness behavior* characterized by the subjective report of physical symptoms, behavioral expression of pain and disability, and the seeking of medical care. The authors proposed that alexithymia may influence organic disease and/or illness behavior through physiological, behavioral, cognitive, or social pathways.

The physiological pathway is believed to operate through the undifferentiated emotion or affect that characterizes alexithymia. Affect is associated with emotional arousal, and because "affect differentiation, elaboration, and regulation is impaired, the arousal remains active, potentially disturbing the autonomic, pituitary-adrenal, and/or immune systems, and eventuating in tissue pathology" (Lumley et al., 1996, p. 507). There is some evidence that alexithymia is associated with higher baseline levels of sympathetic activity. Clinically, higher rates of alexithymia have been found among individuals with hypertension. An example of how alexithymia might operate through social pathways relates to individuals' overly dependent or aloof natures. These attributes would impair social functioning and influence disease indirectly, through physiological pathways. Add the fact that alexithymics are cognitively and behaviorally characterized by disturbed attention toward somatic functioning and poor habits of self-care when alone, and we can begin to see the multifaceted nature of their risk for illness.

Sifneos (1996) believes that there is no point in trying to get at the verbal unconscious of these individuals because their deficit has a neurobiological origin—possibly in terms of disturbances in connections between the limbic system and the neocortex. He recommends leaving treatment to medication. Krystal (1982) echoes the pessimistic view of using dynamic psychotherapy with alexithymic individuals. Trying to provide alexithymic patients with greater awareness of feelings and related body sensations is similar, according to Krystal, to trying to teach someone who is color-blind to perceive color. He postulates that the absence of early mothering experiences in these individuals results in an adult with no symbolic memory of or ability for self-caring and self-soothing actions.

Although dynamic psychotherapy may be inappropriate for alexithymic patients with somatic symptoms, the question remains whether more direct control of the symptoms is possible through somatic awareness intervention. It may be that the ability or inability to experience emotional feeling goes hand in hand with the ability or inability to experience bodily sensations. Still, it is possible, with hard work, to help alexithymics to become more somatically and emotionally aware. The following clinical example of an alexithymic patient with benign unexplained chest pain illustrates the challenge in treating these individuals.

The patient was a 64-year-old retired lawyer who began experiencing severe and unremitting chest and leg pain following retirement. His pain symptoms became noticeable following minor urinary tract surgery. As the symptoms worsened, the patient became increasingly afraid of activity and would remain in bed for long periods of time. Engaging in any form of conversation with his wife or former colleagues made him feel very agitated and tense. His wife had a zest for living, and the more active she became, the more tense and debilitated the patient became. He could not socialize for more than an hour before feeling that he had to leave the situation with worsening chest pain. Prior to retirement, his interests and social activities were all related to his legal firm and business associates. His present daily activities were restricted to a daily walk, with the remainder of the day spent in isolation.

Although unable to connect his chest symptoms to psychological or situational events, he lived with the continuous apprehension that "something bad" was going to happen but he could not describe this apprehension in more specific terms. His chest tightness had became noticeable and problematic once before in his life. During a period of marital crisis, his wife actually left. Eventually she agreed to return, and he maintained that "she was not likely to do this again." His view that his marriage was "okay" was not shared by his wife. She was resigned to remaining in the marriage for companionship but had no desire to seek conjoint therapy.

The patient exhibited all the features of clinical alexithymia. He manifested no awareness of inner emotionality, had poor relationship skills, and displayed no sense of intimacy. At the same time, he felt that he was a caring and loving husband. Conversations with his wife were described in nonemotional terms as "the communication thing," and sex was characterized as "something younger people do." Although he recognized at an intellectual level that marital friction might make his chest tightness worse, he had great difficulty making the necessary emotional connections to himself or to his wife in order to lessen the tightness. In the end he believed that he would feel the chest symptom whether his wife was living with him or not.

Although the patient insisted that his emotional and personal life were "normal like everyone else's," he lived each day with a pervasive fear that something bad was going to happen and that he eventually would not be able to take care of himself. He also continually ruminated whether he was ever going to get better but at the same time he could not identify any emotional or interpersonal issues that needed to be addressed. It is significant that the individual was raised by emotionally controlled parents. Feelings were never expressed or discussed and physical contact between child and parents was not allowed. Thus his pervasive apprehension in adulthood may have had developmental origins in the form of unconscious separation anxiety. Throughout his adult life the anxiety was not an issue, but with aging and retirement psychobiological patterns established in childhood became manifest in the form of chest pain and feelings of insecurity.

Numerous medical and nonmedical treatments had been attempted—all without success. Psychotherapy and marital counseling were described by the patient as "boring, unnecessary, and a waste of time." Efforts at biofeedback were unremarkable. During the training session, the electromyographic (EMG) monitor would show evidence of major chest wall muscle tightness. The patient would glance at the screen, look toward the therapist, and ask, "Am I ever going to get better?" Indeed, it was like trying to teach a color-blind person to see color. The patient was next introduced to diaphragmatic breathing exercises that completely disrupted his natural thoracic breathing style. Although he could not generate evidence of diaphragmatic breathing, he was able to begin to stay relaxed when alone or in the company of others. He also slowly learned to connect situational and interpersonal stress to the worsening of his chest symptoms.

This case illustrates that even individuals who lack emotional awareness and expressiveness are able, with practice, to connect their bodily sensations to psychological events. Although training these patients to focus on somatic sensations is hampered by their general lack of emotional awareness, they are able to slowly acquire an appreciation of the link between feeling and bodily states. Somatic awareness development represents a viable objective for all patients with somatization symptoms.

In summary, it appears essential in our understanding of somatization to retain elements from both the psychodynamic and the amplification perspectives. Whereas the amplification model points to here-and-now verbal influences reflecting how the individual reacts to and copes with bodily symptoms, the traditional psychodynamic model directs attention to personality-/temperament-based symptom coping styles representing unique developmental/early life experiences. The psychodynamic model is especially suited to the identification of long-established coping styles and early formative life events. Understanding these events and coping styles is necessary if we are to be successful in assisting individuals who are unable to immediately benefit from somatic awareness training.

In my view, somatization is a complex systemic and psychobiological process involving cultural, interpersonal, and intrapersonal variables. To further our understanding of the psychobiological processes involved, I will now address the most common somatization symptoms seen in medicine: dizziness, dyspnea, and chest pain. These symptoms collectively account for innumerable visits to family medicine and medical specialists in internal medicine, cardiology, gastroenterology, pulmonology, neurology, and ear–nose–throat specialities. These three symptoms are also the core symptoms of anxiety and anxiety disorders—though paradoxically, their occurrence seldom leads to a direct visit to an anxiety specialist, medical or nonmedical (Kennedy & Schwab, 1997). In the discussion to follow, I present a unitary framework for understanding these symptoms in terms of specific coping styles and maladaptive breathing. The advantage of this approach is that it provides patients and therapist with a somatic focus characterized by slow and deep breathing for managing these conditions. Although the determinants of faulty breathing are multidimensional, interventions that deal with breathing awareness can serve as the internal focus or beacon for bringing the symptom(s) under control.

THE ANXIOUS BODY

Although anxiety is generally discussed in subjective or psychological terms, the word actually has bodily rather than mental origins, coming from the Latin word *angere*, meaning to choke or to strangle. The anxiety condition with the greatest relevance for somatization in medical practice is panic anxiety—which is considered a separate diagnostic category within the fourth edition of the *Diagnostic and Statistical Manual of Mental Disorders* (DSM-IV; American Psychiatric Association, 1994):

> A panic attack is a discrete period in which there is the sudden onset of intense apprehension, fearfulness, or terror, often associated with feelings of impending doom. During these attacks, symptoms such as shortness of breath, palpitations, chest pain or discomfort, choking or smothering sensations, and fear of "going crazy" or losing control are present. (p. 393)

Other somatic symptoms indicative of panic anxiety are nausea, numbness, tingling sensations, and chills or hot flashes. These somatic symptoms correspond to the most common somatization disorders seen in medical practice, indicating that anxiety, whether verbalized or not during symptom presentation, is at the basis of the majority of somatization disorders. These symptoms often occur in a limited fashion, and consequently do not warrant a psychiatric diagnosis of panic disorder. For example, an individual may experience unexplained dizziness and not complain of other bodily and psychological symptoms required for a diagnosis of panic disorder. The absence of obvious psychological precipitants and strategies for management explains why most patients with isolated somatic anxiety symptoms seek further investigation from a variety of medical specialists, including neurologists, cardiologists, gastroenterologists, and ophthalmologists. However, the onset of such symptoms can often be traced to subtle psychological and bodily events—even though they go unnoticed by the patient him/herself.

Panic anxiety is one of the few psychobiological disorders that can be produced within the laboratory. Panic induction is usually achieved through some form of biological provocation, such as inhalation of carbon dioxide. A single breath of 35% CO_2/65% O_2, for example, will generate a variety of bodily sensations, including feelings of breathlessness and suffocation. Patients with panic disorder are vulnerable to the 35% CO_2 challenge but nonanxious volunteers are not. Not all panic-prone individuals respond with panic in this situation, and there is growing evidence that psychological factors involving anticipatory anxiety, uncontrollability, and level of agoraphobia (fear of situations in which escape might be difficult) are more crucial than postulated biological factors. It is often assumed that the main difference in panic responsiveness between panic-prone individuals and controls is the fact that panic-prone persons exhibit heightened sensitivity to otherwise underlying benign physiological changes.

Panic-prone individuals are known to possess a heightened sensitivity to bodily sensations associated with anxiety. Asmundson, Norton, Wilson, and Sandler (1994) had college students complete a questionnaire that assesses fear of anxiety symptoms. The questionnaire data were used to form groups based on the degree of self-reported anxiety sensitivity. Next, subjects were asked to engage in forced hyperventilation by breathing at a rate of 30 cycles per minute. Heart rate was measured throughout the hyperventilation period. Subjects were also asked to rate the intensity of physical and cognitive symptoms experienced during the hyperventilation challenge. The subjects in the high anxiety–sensitive group rated all the panic symptoms as being more severe than the low anxiety–sensitive group. The groups did not differ in terms of their observed heart rates. Studies that find psychological differences but no physiological differences between panic-prone individuals and controls are interpreted as showing that the main determinant of the panic experience is psychological rather than physiological; that is, panickers are simply "overreacting to" or "misinterpreting" normal physiological events. There is an element of misinterpretation in reading their bodies by panic sufferers, but the misinterpretation is understandable if one has no other explanation for the symptoms that are occurring. It would be a mistake, however, to conclude, on the basis of lack of observed increases in heart rate or some other physiological index, that there are no significant bodily events taking place. More often than not, there is a physiological substrate accounting for the bodily sensations being experienced. This substrate needs to be recognized by the panic sufferer before the symptoms can be effectively managed. There is more going on than faulty thinking.

The heavy emphasis in psychology on cognitive determinants of panic anxiety has its origins in the writings of Aaron Beck. In *Anxiety Disorders and Phobias,* Beck and Emery (1985) described the case of a 40-year-old man who had gone on a skiing trip and while skiing began to experience shortness of breath, perspiration, faintness, and body weakness. He had difficulty focusing and eventually was removed from the slopes via stretcher and rushed to the hospital. Nothing abnormal was found and he received the diagnosis of acute anxiety attack. The man was an experienced skier who had in the past simply "skied through" similar body symptoms (chest pain, feeling cold, being sweaty). Why the difference this time? According to Beck and Emery, some cognitive circumstance led him to interpret these previously benign exercise sensations as having life-threatening significance. He had recently lost a brother due to heart attack and must have thought, "If it could happen to my brother, it could happen to me. . . . " The skier may indeed have been questioning his mortality. But I doubt very much that the frightening body sensations that he experienced were in fact similar to those occurring under an exercise state. On this day, his body and mind were likely triggered into a state of panic; consequently, he was correct in identifying within himself a condition that was different from the sensations resulting from normal exercise. We must be careful not to assume that nothing of significance was happening within his body.

Beck's theoretical and clinical emphasis on the cognitive aspects of anxiety reflected in large part his belief that treatment had become too dependent on the chemical control of the physical symptoms of anxiety. Yet he remained acutely aware that anxiety has powerful biological origins, and he wrote at length of the psychobiological nature of a primitive "fight–flight–freeze" reaction at the basis of many occurrences of anxiety episodes. The significance of the somatic aspects of anxiety is reflected in the content of the Beck Anxiety Inventory (BAI; Beck & Steer, 1990). The BAI contains 21 items, with 6 items reflecting cognitive symptoms (e.g., fear of the worst happening, scared, terrified) and the remaining 14 items reflecting somatic symptoms (e.g., feelings of choking, dizzy or lightheaded, face flushed).

A cluster analysis of the inventory by Beck and Steer (1990) identified four groups of symptoms. The four clusters of BAI symptoms were based on a large sample of outpatients with anxiety disorders. The dominant cluster is called "neurophysiological" and contains symptoms associated with feeling dizzy, faint, numb, and wobbly in the legs. The second cluster is characterized by subjective symptoms such as fear of the worst happening, fear of losing control, being terrified, and being unable to relax. The first two symptoms are consistent with the cognitive fear-of-fear hypothesis. The third cluster contains a mixture of cardiovascular (heart pounding), respiratory (difficulty breathing, sensations of choking), and subjective (fear of dying) symptoms. The symptoms "feelings of choking," "difficulty breathing," and "pounding heart" are extremely prevalent across anxiety disorders. Panic disorder symptoms of chest pain and/or chest tightness were not included in the questionnaire, though their inclusion might have provided evidence for a distinct respiratory/chest pain symptom cluster. The fourth cluster is characterized by autonomic symptoms of feeling hot, sweaty, and flushed, and to a lesser extent feeling abdominal discomfort.

A later report by Beck, Steer, and Beck (1993) demonstrated that three, rather than four, factors characterize the responses of anxiety patients to the BAI. In this study the autonomic factor identified in the original study loads on the neurophysiological factor. Cox, Cohen, Direnfeld, and Swinson (1996) administered the BAI to a large sample of panic disorder patients and identified three factors with the same content as the factors identified by Beck and colleagues. Cox et al. labeled their factors "dizziness," to correspond to neurophysiological; "cardiorespiratory," to correspond to panic; and "catastrophic cognitions/fear" to correspond to subjective.

Similar clusters of bodily and subjective symptoms have been identified in nonclinical populations, indicating that somatic patterning is present in anxious individuals prior to clinical symptom development. My colleagues and I (Egger, Bakal, & Fung, 1998) conducted a similar unpublished cluster analysis of the BAI based on the responses of 527 college students. The questionnaire was administered as part of a larger study dealing with somatic ratings of anxiety and depression. The three BAI college student clusters were quite similar to the three-factor solutions obtained from anxiety patients. The finding is important for theories of anxiety and somatization. Current theories place inordinate emphasis on the catastrophic aspects of anxiety and ignore the countless patients who present to medical clinics in the absence of subjective fear and distress. Current theories of anxiety, whether psychological, biological, or psychobiological do not address individual differences in subjective and/or physical symptom development. They do not explain, for example, why one individual presents primarily with unexplained dizziness with little or no subjective fear and another individual presents with chest tightness and difficulty breathing and fears of going crazy.

The observation that bodily anxiety symptoms cluster into neurophysiological and panic groupings is especially important for understanding the different forms of expression of bodily anxiety in medical patients. Patients with unexplained dizziness, for example, often seek out neurologists because of their fear of serious disease such as multiple sclerosis, while those with persistent respiratory and chest symptoms may seek out examination by a cardiologist.

I will now take a closer look at the main symptoms from the two somatic factors, dizziness from the neurophysiological factor and difficulty breathing from the panic factor. Difficulty breathing is discussed under the heading of dyspnea (shortness of breath) and chest pain. We will see that although the subjective and situational determinants may be quite different for dizziness and breathing symptoms, both symptoms may also share similar physiological mechanisms, albeit different in direction. I will also examine the common clinical situation in which individuals present with somatic symptoms but show little or no sign of subjective distress.

Unexplained Dizziness

Unexplained sensations of dizziness as well as wobbliness, unsteadiness, and feeling faint are some of the most frequently reported somatization symptoms experienced by patients. The dizziness experienced by somatizing patients is not associated with a rotating sensation or vertigo, indicative of vestibular dysfunction. It is more nonspecific in experience, such that patients with this symptom have difficulty putting into words the sensations they are experiencing. Common descriptors include "lightheadedness," "feeling detached," and "fuzziness." Dyspnea and chest pain are somatic symptoms that sometimes co-occur with dizziness and sometimes do not.

Dizziness episodes sometimes occur during periods of relaxation or inactivity and resemble the state of relaxation-induced anxiety (Heide & Borkovec, 1984). Fewtrell and O'Connor (1988) provided an example of a teacher who was prone to dizzy bouts on relaxing weekends and holidays, but never experienced these in the classroom. They proposed that abrupt arousal shifts, upward or downward may provoke dizziness.

Some instances of dizziness may be experienced as a form of depersonalization. Fewtrell and O'Connor (1988) defined "depersonalization" as an unpleasant change in the quality of consciousness in which there is a reduction of intensity of feeling, accompanied by a curious change of self-awareness. Slater and Roth (1969) described depersonalization phenomena as a form of "constriction of consciousness" that is activated by severe anxiety and that serves to attenuate the effects of anxiety on behavior. Depersonalization serves, then, to protect the individual during periods of intolerable distress. To illustrate the relationship between fear, anxiety, and depersonalization, they related an incident of a psychiatrist who was involved in a traffic accident on his way to work:

> The man in question was driving at some speed on a wet road surface and as he cornered fast the car skidded. He immediately experienced a dream-like detachment and found himself steering mechanically and aware of his actions as if he were contemplating some unfortunate victim from a distance. After spinning round several times and narrowly avoiding oncoming traffic, the car finally came to a halt facing in the opposite direction. The driver felt quite calm but when by-standers spoke to him their voices seemed muffled and the surrounding countryside appeared still, remote and unreal. His own voice sounded unfamiliar. He drove on feeling quite calm, arrived at his clinic and rang for his first patient. As the patient entered the psychiatrist's depersonalization suddenly lifted and he became quite aware that he was perspiring and trembling severely and his heart was pounding at a rapid rate. (pp. 122–123)

Fewtrell and O'Connor hypothesize that dizziness and depersonalization may be phenomenologically identical and may reflect variation in patients' choice of semantics in describing the same perceptual disturbance.

Clinical occurrences of dizziness in public settings first led to the identification of agoraphobia as an anxiety disorder. In 1870 Benedikt reported a clinical state he called *Platzschwindel,* which means "dizziness in public places." This observation was followed by Westphal's publication a year later using the term "agoraphobia" for the same phenomenon (Boyd & Crump, 1991). Westphal presented the cases of three men who had a strong fear of crossing open spaces. One individual experienced both dizziness and heart palpitations; the second individual described feeling of heat beginning in the lower part of the abdomen and rising toward the head, heart palpitations, tremor, and a feeling of bewilderment; and the third individual felt chest tightness in the region of the heart, followed by heat sensations in the face and feelings of derealization. All patients reported no identifiable reason for their fear, and all were able to benefit from having someone accompany them and/or a drink of alcohol prior to entering the open space. Westphal noted that dizziness was a common symptom of these individuals, and he believed that its origins were purely cerebral or mental.

Dizziness seems to occur more frequently in individuals who have a fear of or preoccupation with having to cope in public, while shortness of breath and chest pain seem to be reported more frequently when the individual is alone at home and has a fear of impending heart attack. Ottaviani and Beck (1987) asked subjects to recall the thoughts and images that were present during an episode of panic and also to indicate the situational context in which the attack occurred. The qualitative data they collected suggested that subjects reported dizziness and disorientation sensations when their attacks occurred in public situations (e.g., shopping, caught in a crowd, talking to a boss) and chest pain and shortness of breath sensations when their attacks occurred in private, usually at home. There was, however, considerable overlap of the two categories of symptoms. These were retrospective and uncontrolled accounts, making it impossible to know the degree to which dizziness and dyspnea occurred together but were noticed differently depending on the patient's situational circumstance.

A connection between fear of social situations and dizziness is suggested in a study by Telch, Brouillard, Telch, Agras, and Taylor (1989). They observed that the main symptoms that differentiated panic disorder patients with agoraphobia from panic disorder patients without agoraphobia were feeling faint and dizziness. A number of cognitive symptoms related to social embarrassment and loss of control also differentiated the two groups, but the physical symptom of dizziness most clearly separated the groups in terms of their situational avoidance. It appears that the demands of certain social situations bring about physiological changes that operate outside of awareness, leading to the symptom of dizziness. My personal hypothesis is that these individuals engage in extremely shallow breathing punctuated by periods of complete absence of breath that eventually initiates a state of hyperventilation followed by dizziness. Similar restricted breathing occurs in patients who are at risk for falling. I have seen many elderly patients who engage in walking and other physical activities as if they are swimming underwater—taking a gulp of air, holding their breath, and "going for it." Invariably, they have no awareness that they are breath holding in this fashion. This style of breathing is especially prevalent if they have already fallen, broken a leg or hip, and have a fear of falling again.

Dizziness leading to loss of consciousness and postural tone is called "syncope" (Linzer et al., 1991). The loss of consciousness is believed to result from anxiety-generated sympathetic tone followed by a homeostatic parasympathetic response with associated bradycardia and hypotension. Like agoraphobics, these individuals often develop a fear of fainting and consequent functional impairment. Syncope often leads to interference with daily activities, driving, employment, and interpersonal relationships. There is no awareness of bodily changes prior to the loss of consciousness:

> A 72-year-old patient was admitted to hospital with long-standing pain secondary to Mellaril. The majority of pain occurred around the perineal region and the mouth and gums. The individual had

received a diagnosis of posttraumatic stress disorder (PTSD) during World War II and had been receiving anxiolytic and antipsychotic medications for over 40 years. He had experienced numerous episodes of being angry with the medical system for prescribing phenothiazines. He was admitted to a rehabilitation unit for the purpose of withdrawing him from phenothiazines and benzodiazepines. The patient had one activity for reducing pain: watching TV. One evening he was having difficulty sleeping so he went to the TV room to watch late night shows. After an hour he began to sweat and decided to make his way to bed. On the way he lost consciousness and fell to the floor. He insisted, after the episode, that he could recall no reason for the event. This is a common observation of syncope patients in that they all believe that the episodes are unexplained, even though there is often evidence of emotional tension or apprehension within the period prior to an episode. This particular patient was extremely sensitive to perceived staff criticism of his actions and on this night he was watching TV in the same room that the night staff used for their coffee breaks. The awareness that he was preventing the staff from using the room may have generated anxiety, although he never acknowledged that this was the case.

The syncope patient also noted the presence of chest pain during his dizziness; he felt as if "I could not open my lungs up." This indicates that there may be a respiratory and/or ventilatory component to syncope, the extent of which is unknown. It is quite possible that the experiences of dizziness and chest symptoms, although not necessarily perceived as occurring together, may have their origins in breathing changes associated with shallow breathing and increased chest wall muscle tone. Shortness of breath and dizziness are both associated with hyperventilation (Drachman & Hart, 1972). Hyperventilation is known to lead to vasoconstriction of the cerebral vasculature and accompanying dizziness and depersonalization.

Dyspnea and Chest Pain

Dyspnea and chest pain/tightness, like dizziness, represent some of the most common somatic symptoms seen in medical practice. Dyspnea or breathlessness has received the most attention in the anxiety literature because of its significance to ventilatory explanations of panic disorder. Chest pain is also a very common symptom reported in surveys of symptoms in the general population and those in ambulatory care. The pain may be located in any part of the thorax and can be experienced as sharp and stabbing pain or as cramplike. The detection of a physical explanation for the pain has observed to be as low as 11% of patients presenting at an internal medicine clinic (Kroenke & Mangelsdorff, 1989). It is not easy to separate the experiences of chest pain due to cardiac versus noncardiac causes. Cardiologists describe coronary pain or angina as a heaviness, a burning, a pressure, or a squeezing sensation below the sternum. The sensation is often described more as a discomfort than pain and can radiate up to the left shoulder and down the left arm and sometimes extend to the lower jaw. Angina pain is precipitated by exertion and promptly relieved by rest or nitroglycerin. The diagnostic difficulty is that pain that is not due to angina can at times exhibit the same characteristics as pain indicative of a developing heart attack.

Research is required to determine how the sensory characteristics of benign chest pain differ from those of angina. An acute myocardial infarction or heart attack requires immediate medical attention. It is known that mortality can be reduced by as much as 50% if treatment is initiated within 1 hour of the onset of symptoms (Dracup et al., 1995). Thus, one could be at great risk by ignoring chest sensations or by believing that chest sensations are benign in origin when in fact they are not. Even medical experts may not be able to differentiate benign chest pain from an impending heart attack. According to Julian (1996), who undertook a survey of the behavior of 10 world-renowned cardiologists who had heart attacks, on average, they delayed seeking help for 48 hours, presumably on the assumption that the pain they were experiencing was not indicative of heart failure.

But our concern is with individuals who experience chest pain in the absence of coronary disease. Follow-up studies have shown that patients with chest pain and normal coronary arteries continue to exhibit high levels of illness behavior (e.g., restrictions in daily living, emotional distress, continued use of medical resources) even though they have repeatedly been told that they do not have heart disease (Bass, 1992). Even if the patients accept the diagnosis of benign chest pain, they are left to wonder what is causing the pain. In the past, symptoms of dyspnea and chest tightness were assumed to invariably have a cardiac origin. In the 1800s benign chest symptoms were referred to as "irritable heart syndrome," "Da Costa's syndrome," "soldier's heart," and "effort syndrome"; in all cases, the symptoms experienced were attributed to irritability or abnormal reaction of the heart to exertion (Skerritt, 1983). In the early 1900s the syndrome of chest pain and shortness of breath was believed to have unspecified nervous rather than cardiac origin.

Current research is examining unexplained chest pain as a variant of panic disorder and looking toward ventilatory, respiratory, or some ventilatory–respiratory explanation for the symptoms. Ventilatory models deal primarily with central neurophysiological mechanisms (e.g., brainstem chemoreceptors) that regulate breathing, while respiratory models focus more on the psychophysiological variables involved in breathing. The leading advocate of the ventilatory explanation of dyspnea and other chest symptoms is Klein (1993). He is particularly interested in these symptoms' unique contribution to panic anxiety. He believes that ventilatory symptoms such as changes in minute ventilation are specific to panic anxiety, while cardiac symptoms (palpitations) can be found with both panic disorder and generalized anxiety patients. Klein developed the hyperventilation theory of panic anxiety with the postulation of a biological *suffocation alarm system*. He hypothesized that individuals who are susceptible to panic disorder possess a derangement of the suffocation centers of the brain. He surmises that our brain naturally has a way of sounding an alarm if we are being suffocated, and that in some people this regulatory thermostat may have an incorrectly low threshold, such that alarm bells go off intermittently, causing the person to gasp for air. Breathlessness is, in Klein's view, a preliminary phase of panic that initiates hyperventilation. Breathlessness itself is initiated by the suffocation alarm, that is, an internal or endogenous danger signal. The perception of the increased drive to breathe is then assumed to result in misattribution to catastrophic causes such as heart attack.

It is critical to know what the physiological determinants of benign chest pain are. After all, the pain is real and persistent and cannot simply be attributed to overconcern, misattribution, or amplification. There is a good possibility that chest pain and breathlessness might be associated with heightened activity of muscles in the chest wall. This belief is based on some observations made of panic sufferers with chest tightness during a laboratory CO_2 provocation study (Lynch, Bakal, Whitelaw, & Fung, 1991). The study was designed to examine Klein's hypothesis that panic sufferers possess an overly sensitive suffocation alarm system and overreact (as evidenced by greater than normal changes in heart rate and depth of breathing) when exposed to different concentrations of CO_2 inhalations. As part of the study, surface electromyographic (EMG) activity was recorded from the sternum region of the chest simply to see if there might be a peripheral musculoskeletal correlate of the symptoms of chest tightness, pressure, and/or heaviness. The panic disorder subjects were divided on the basis of how anxious or "panicky" they became during the course of the experiment, as determined by several administrations of a 10-point Likert scale. Although there were no differences in the breathing parameters, there were significant differences in chest EMG, with the high anxious panic subjects exhibiting the greatest activity. Heightened chest muscle activity was observed only in the panic disorder subjects who were also showing evidence of anxiety and/or panic in response to the CO_2 challenge. The observations of sustained chest wall EMG activity were made during periods of end expiration and were therefore indicative of inspiratory effort that was maintained throughout the whole breathing cycle. Thus, the muscles were holding the chest in a tonic fashion at a volume higher than its relaxed volume, plus making repeated inspiratory efforts to increase volume further for each breath. Such activity is abnormal and serves no physiological purpose.

We could not determine whether the heightened chest EMG activity was chronic in nature or specific to the experimental situation. Our suspicion is that the activity was specific to the situation and that the pulmonary laboratory proved to be highly provoking for the more severe agoraphobic panic disorder patients. The hallmark characteristic of agoraphobic avoidance is "the fear of being in places or situations from which escape might be difficult (or embarrassing) or in which help might not be available in the event of having a Panic Attack or panic-like symptoms" (American Psychiatric Association, 1994, p. 396). Laboratory situations, from this definition, should be especially panic provoking for agoraphobic individuals. In the situation reported above, subjects were attached to numerous transducers and were required to wear an air-flow face mask and a nose-clip for periods of up to 1 hour. The observed panic reactions and heightened chest wall muscle activity had more to do with situational constraint than the activation of brainstem chemoreceptors from inhaled CO_2.

Knowing that chest wall muscle activity is a determinant of the pain experienced is important in helping individuals understand their symptom. Although simply saying, "Mr. Jones, your chest pain is due not to heart disease, but rather to overstretched chest wall muscles resulting from stress and worry" is not likely to resolve the symptom, it is one step better than saying, "The cardiac tests are normal so there is nothing to worry about." Patient awareness that the bodily sensations are associated with breathing and muscle can give the sufferer a far less "catastrophic" view of their origin. Now the challenge becomes one of fostering an experiential connectedness of chest wall sensations and the other dimensions of conscious experience related to emotional and interpersonal living.

PHYSICAL SYMPTOMS
WITHOUT SUBJECTIVE DISTRESS

We have seen that not all patients who present with somatic symptoms present with psychological symptoms. In actuality, there are likely to be as many individuals who experience somatic symptoms and who deny the existence of psychological distress as individuals who present with both somatic and psychological distress. Outside of concepts like alexithymia, psychological theories of somatic symptoms have generally ignored these individuals, preferring instead to concentrate on those who verbalize excessively or inappropriately about their somatic condition. We need to learn much more about the large number of individuals who experience somatic symptoms in the absence of psychological distress.

Many patients seen in hospital clinics present with somatic symptoms in the absence of psychological concerns but have symptoms with a psychobiological origin. Unfortunately, these individuals are seldom properly managed and their untreated condition leads to endless investigations and prescriptions for treatment that are often ineffective. Too often health professionals mistakenly assume that if the subjective fear or anxiety is not experienced in the presence of a somatic symptom such as dizziness or chest pain, the underlying cause must be neurological or physiological. However, the cause can readily be psychobiological and within the individual's awareness and control.

Kushner, Beitman, and Beck (1989) noted that only half of a sample of chest pain cardiology patients with normal or near normal coronary arteries verbalized anxiety, whereas the other half of the sample did not verbalize significant anxiety. Kushner and Beitman (1990) used these observations to describe a clinical condition that they labeled *nonfearful panic disorder*. Nonfearful panic disorder captures a clinical condition in which affected individuals experience attacks or episodes of symptoms that meet criteria for the psychiatric diagnosis of panic disorder (i.e., in terms of number, type, and frequency of symptoms) but do not include the diagnostic cognitive symptoms involving feelings of fear, fear of losing control, or fear of going crazy. Patients with nonfearful panic disorder typically present for treatment to medical clinics specializing in the bodily symptom in which they are experiencing their symptoms. Thus they may present as cardiology patients, as gastrointestinal patients, as neurology patients, or as simply primary care patients. In many instances they have undergone a long history of diagnostic procedures that were negative in outcome:

One of these cases, for example, was a 31 yr. old surgeon referred by his neurologist for a psychiatric evaluation because of attacks of near syncope which had been occurring for 6 months, chiefly at the beginning of difficult vascular operations. The patient had no prior psychiatric history and stated that he did not feel that he needed psychiatric consultation but admitted to increasing stress at work with the loss of his new partner approx. 10 months before this evaluation. The patient also admitted to having lost a patient in surgery for the first time in his career approx. 8 months prior to the evaluation and 1 month prior to the onset of his recurrent near syncopal episodes. He related a family history of depression and anxiety attacks in his mother. The patient, who described himself as a perfectionist, said that his father had died in surgery approx. 1 yr. before the patient entered medical school. These episodes were described as feeling like "lights were going out." He also felt like he was having difficulty breathing during that time and said that he began to sweat all over. He said that he did not experience anxiety during the episodes although he was beginning to feel worried when entering the operating room about having another attack and had cut back on his operating schedule. (Kushner & Beitman, 1990, p. 473)

Some experts believe that panic disorder has its initial onset in the form of somatic symptoms and then evolves to include cognitive symptoms associated with catastrophic thinking (Rosenbaum, 1987). Nonpatients and student samples in the community with a history of panic attacks report a low incidence of cognitive panic symptoms. However, the difference between panic patients without cognitive symptoms and those with cognitive symptoms may have less to do with panic severity and more to do with differences in subjective coping styles. For individuals who lack subjective anxiety, wearing feelings "on one's sleeve" is out of keeping with their controlled emotional style, such that anxiety may manifest only at the somatic level. Such individuals, in exhibiting physiological response to threat, may simply not experience the subjective anxiety seen in a characteristic panic reaction.

Nonfearful panic disorder is likely characterized by a different psychophysiological profile from the profile that occurs during the classic panic reaction. Classic panic reactions are characterized by intense subjective fear and rapid increases in heart rate, increases in breathing rate, and shortness of breath. The assumption behind nonfearful panic disorder is that everything remains the same, minus the subjective fear. This may not be the case. Psychophysiological data from a case study (Bakal, Fung, & Hesson, 1996) suggest that nonfearful panic sufferers may respond quite differently from regular panic sufferers at the physiological as well as at the subjective levels.

The case study involved a 36-year-old unemployed engineer who began experiencing severe dizziness at a time when business and marital problems became overwhelming. The dizziness proved to have no organic cause and was not associated with vertigo or syncope. He described the dizziness as "lightheadedness," "faintness," and "fogginess." The dizziness symptom was unresponsive to both antidepressant and anxiolytic medication. Daily charting of the dizziness revealed no obvious psychological or situational triggers, and the symptom would often appear "out of the blue." A psychiatric interview revealed no fear of dying or losing control during the dizziness episodes. There was no evidence of blood phobia, social phobia, or agoraphobia.

The patient had agreed to participate in a research study dealing with panic provocation under laboratory conditions. The panic provocation induction procedure involved a single breath inhalation of 35% CO_2. The procedure consisted of coaching the subject to exhale all air from his lungs followed by a single deep inhalation of 35% CO_2 gas mixture through a mouthpiece apparatus and holding the breath for 5 seconds. The inhalation is associated with an intense feeling of suffocation and, in the case of typical panic sufferers, accompanying autonomic arousal and subjective distress. Increases in respiration rate, heart rate, and catastrophic thinking are commonly reported by panic sufferers following a single breath of 35% CO_2.

This individual did not show a response profile resembling that of panic disorder patients. First, there was no evidence of autonomic arousal. His respiration rate remained unchanged and his heart rate dropped dramatically from a baseline average of 67 beats per minute to 43 beats per minute following the inhalation. This reaction was surprising given that 35% CO_2 inhalation creates a very strong bodily need to "blow off" the excess CO_2. Even nonanxious individuals exhibit a brief increase in breathing rate, not the observed decrease in heart rate. This patient reported little or no fear and appeared to be trying to remain "in control" throughout the provocation. He described experiencing a "field of red" for a few seconds and an intense sense of gasping for air. There was no self-reported fear although he acknowledged a fleeting sense of losing control.

Somatic awareness varies across individuals with a number of different physical symptoms. The lack of awareness can have serious consequences. Angina pectoris (pain and constriction about the heart) is the most common symptom of myocardial ischemia. Myocardial ischemia occurs when the oxygen requirement of the cardiac muscle exceeds its supply. Ischemia may be associated with painful sensations or it may not. In patients with coronary artery disease, the majority of out-of-hospital ischemic episodes are asymptomatic or without bodily sensation. It is difficult to know why chest pain symptoms sometimes accompany ischemic episodes and sometimes do not. Some symptomatic patients tend to complain of chest pain early in the course of ischemic episodes, even if their symptoms are relatively mild, whereas others endure prolonged ischemia before reporting any symptoms. Freedland et al. (1990) identified a group of patients with chest pain and reversible myocardial ischemia and a group of patients with silent ischemia during an exercise stress test. At the start of the exercise patients were instructed to report any chest discomfort, fatigue, or other symptoms. All patients were asked to report the time at which they expected to be able to continue exercising only one more minute. The onset of chest pain was the most common reason given by symptomatic patients as the reason for terminating the stress test. The most common reason given by the asymptomatic patients was fatigue.

There were no significant differences between the groups with respect to total exercise duration or time from onset of electrocardiograph indications of ischemia to the end of exercise. The asymptomatic group scored significantly lower on a revised Autonomic Perception Questionnaire (APQ; Mandler, Mandler, & Uviller, 1958). The APQ, as noted in the opening chapter, assesses how frequently a respondent perceives sensations associated with autonomic nervous system activity. The standard APQ is limited to sensations that occur when the individual is anxious. In this study it was modified to include the perception of autonomic and other general bodily sensations. The silent ischemics scored much lower than the symptomatic patients. The researchers hypothesized that since the markedly lower APQ scores of the asymptomatic patients were based not just on cardiac sensations but on bodily sensations in general, this group might be characterized by an absence of awareness of bodily sensations of any origin. Other research suggests that asymptomatic ischemia patients exhibit a reduced sensitivity to noncardiac painful stimuli (Droste, Greenlee, & Roskamm, 1986).

Frasure-Smith (1987) presented data showing a strong inverse relationship between the report of bodily symptoms and degree of blockage in coronary arteries as measured by coronary catheterization. The study measured body awareness in terms of the degree to which subjects experienced a number of noncardiac bodily symptoms during the past week. The symptoms were similar to those assessed by the BAI and included blurring of vision, stomach churning, and feeling hot all over. What motivated the study was the clinical observation that patients with severe blockages of the heart often seem to avoid seeking medical attention until the disease progresses, while, conversely, individuals with little or no blockage often present early in the process. Of medical concern are those individuals who seem to not experience or to deny early warning symptoms such as chest pain. The author speculated that these men may also be low in terms of somatic awareness. The results provided strong support for this hypothesis: subjects with no vessels blocked had mean somatic perception scores of 10.7, with 1 vessel blocked scores of 6.0, with two vessels blocked scores of 3.8, and with 3 or 4 vessels blocked scores of 3.3. Thus, the greater the blockage, the lower the number of symptoms reported.

The Frasure-Smith study did not assess symptoms directly related to angina and chest pain. Therefore it is unknown whether the groups differed in terms of perception of bodily symptoms related to their disease or simply differed in terms of levels of hypochondriasis. The latter interpretation is clearly plausible given that the low somatic perception scores of the individuals with blocked vessels resembled the scores provided by normals. It is possible, then, that there is no relationship between lack of bodily awareness and severity of coronary artery disease. There is, however, growing evidence that individuals with heart disease need to take precautions to minimize the impact of psychological stress on their hearts. Jiang et al. (1996) demonstrated that individuals with documented coronary artery disease who reacted with signs of myocardial ischemia during laboratory mental stress induction procedures showed increased likelihood of adverse cardiac events during a 2- to 5-year follow-up period.

A more recent comparison of silent versus symptomatic myocardial ischemia patients reported a different psychological profile for the two groups (Torosian, Lumley, Pickard, & Ketterer, 1997). A sample of 102 individuals (78 men, 24 women) underwent treadmill stress testing. Sixty-eight subjects were asymptomatic during the procedure and 34 subjects showed symptoms of ischemia. The symptoms considered diagnostic of ischemia included tightness, pressure, or fullness in the chest; discomfort radiating to the jaw, arms, or upper back; or anginal symptoms that subjects reported to be typical for them. The subjects with silent ischemia exhibited greater externally oriented thinking (as measured by an alexithymia questionnaire), lower somatosensory amplification, and a higher degree of anger control than the symptomatic subjects. This study also reported that the two groups did not differ in terms of their cardiac assessments, that is, the presence and extent of medically assessed ischemia. The observed psychological variables appeared to be operating independent of medical variables associated with cardiac disease. This does not mean that the pain and associated symptoms experienced by the symptomatic group are without physiological basis. It does suggest, however, that other physiological variables, such as chest wall muscle activity, should be considered. This study represents one of a growing number that demonstrate that there are very significant individual differences operating in the way individuals experience bodily sensations associated with physiological symptom development. These differences have major implications for clinical management. Torosian et al. (1997) noted that the lack of bodily symptom experience or recognition may "interfere with taking preventive actions, seeking treatment, or accurately describing one's symptoms to a health care professional" (p. 123). The psychological profile accompanying the lack of symptom recognition also makes somatic awareness as a therapeutic intervention more difficult to achieve.

Another example of differences in bodily perception of symptom onset with major clinical implications is found with asthmatics. Although asthma is widely regarded as a physical illness in need of medical treatment, isolated evidence indicates that some asthmatics can utilize bodily information to prevent attacks as well as to lessen the severity of their asthmatic episodes. Thus I find it surprising that bodily awareness has not attained mainstream intervention status in the management of asthma.

During an asthmatic episode, breathing is impeded by the constriction of airway muscles and the swelling of mucous membranes and other tissues that line the airways, and by the accumulation of mucous in the airways. Asthmatic attacks are described as mild, moderate, or severe (status asthmaticus; Weiss, 1994).

> The typical symptoms of asthma include sensations of tightness in the chest, air hunger, and an inability to breathe without deliberate, even great, effort. The patient's struggle to inhale is marked by a hunched-over posture, hands pressed against a table top, chair back or other surface (as if to get leverage in the effort to breathe), shoulders drawn up and back and chest heaving. Associated with the problem in breathing *in* is the patient's inability to *exhale* normally, which results in air being trapped in the lungs, thus reducing *vital capacity* [the maximum volume of air that can be moved in and out of the lung] to breathe in and out. Paradoxically, the harder patients try to breathe, the more resistance they may feel, the more frightened they may become, and the harder they may try. (Weiss, 1994, p. 206)

Many asthmatic individuals fail to recognize both the presence of anxiety within themselves and early changes in airflow obstruction (Yellowlees & Kalucy, 1990). Lack of awareness of symptom onset has been linked to occurrences of fatal asthmatic attacks in both children and adults (Fritz, Rubinstein, & Lewiston, 1987). Developing dyspnea in the early stages of the asthmatic attack is not perceived by a good percentage of asthmatic individuals. Heim, Blaser, and Waidelich (1972) defined dyspnea as "the unpleasant feeling of difficulty or inability to breathe based on the perception of real, threatened, or fantasied impairment of ventilation" (p. 406). They provide this broad definition to illustrate that dyspnea is similar to pain in that it involves both the *perception of* and the *reaction to* bodily sensations. In their experiment they exposed asthmatics and other groups to carbachol, a bronchoconstrictive agent designed to induce dyspnea. Following the carbachol inhalation, the asthmatic subjects were required to rate their breathlessness. This rating was compared with an objective measure of airway resistance obtained with a plethysmograph. The researchers then devised a subjective difference score (SDS) for each subject to express the difference in rank between subjective ratings of dyspnea and objective findings. A positive SDS meant that the subject demonstrated objective evidence of dyspnea in the absence of subjective evidence, while a negative SDS meant that the subject rated the subjective experience of dyspnea as greater than what was observed with the airway resistance measure.

Four of 22 patients showed positive SDSs greater than 20, indicating that they were not reporting dyspnea in spite of reduced airway resistance. These "minimizers" presented themselves during a separate clinical interview as being in control of their feelings, efficient, and highly ethical in manner. Eight of 22 patients had SDSs greater than 20, which indicates that a large number of asthmatics may be overreacting to perceived airway resistance. The authors describe these individuals as being both anxious and hypochondriacal.

The most frequent bodily sensation of dyspnea reported by all asthmatics is generally "tightness of breath." This sensation needs further investigation in terms of its potential as a bodily cue for initiating somatic awareness strategies designed to relax the chest wall and reduce respiration rate during a developing asthmatic episode. There is also a need for the study of the role of individual differences in determining somatic awareness across asthma sufferers. It appears that just as many asthmatic individuals overreport body sensations as underreport body sensations, and both extremes can exacerbate the overall illness condition.

I have reviewed evidence that indicates that the major somatization symptoms seen in medical practice closely resemble the somatic symptom groupings observed in anxiety patients. The splitting of bodily symptoms into neurophysiological and panic categories, as well as the inclusion of the subjective domain, represents an important beginning in organizing the diverse presentations of somatic symptoms seen in clinical practice. Further research is needed to determine the possible existence of groupings across the three symptom domains. Kushner et al. (1990), for example, found evidence for a group of cardiac patients who present with no subjective symptoms. We need to determine the similarities and differences of these patients, in terms of their psychological and physiological reactions, to patients who complain primarily of dizziness or other specific symptoms. The young man with unexplained dizziness and complete lack of subjective anxiety who responded to a panic induction procedure with a psychophysiological profile quite different from the profile exhibited in the classic panic reaction illustrates the dramatic nature of individual differences that may occur.

CULTURAL VARIATION

The degree of somatic symptom variation is likely even greater *across* cultures than it is *within* cultures. Few studies have examined how individuals differ across cultures in their presentation of somatic and subjective anxiety symptoms. We have preliminary data that compared the responses of a sample of North American undergraduate students to the BAI with a sample of responses from Arab students (from the United Arab Emirates) to the same questionnaire. The results revealed that the different student cultures were both similar and dissimilar in their responses to the BAI. A three-factor analysis of their responses revealed two factors that were similar in content and one factor that was dissimilar in content to the three factors identified in a North American college student sample. The Arab students resembled the North American students in terms of the neurophysiological and subjective symptom clusters, but they were distinct with respect to the panic factor. The panic factor in North American studies generally consists of fear of dying and cardiorespiratory symptoms involving heart pounding, feelings of choking, and difficulty breathing. In the Arab student sample, the panic factor consisted of fear of dying and temperature symptoms of sweating, face flushing, and feeling hot. The heat symptoms were endorsed with the clear understanding that they were being endorsed in reference to anxiety rather than to external air temperature. Arab psychiatrists have long observed that heat symptoms are very common in generalized anxiety disorder and panic disorder. What is unknown is whether different physiological response systems are also at work across the two cultures.

Multicultural research concerning somatic awareness would shed important information on how different cultures incorporate the body into feelings of health and well-being. We should not overlook the fact that language reflects both conscious and unconscious values, beliefs, and worldviews of the people using it. Thus bodily related words in one culture may have quite different contextual meanings than bodily related words used in another culture. The Chinese, for example, have a rich vocabulary of words and phrases for describing bodily related experiences. For the Chinese, bodily experiences are central to understanding oneself and others. The body is capable of thinking, feeling, and experiencing. The expression *ti hui* means to empathize and is often expressed as the ability to understand with the body alone, without words. The expression *ti yan* means that to truly understand, you must experience with your own body. For the Chinese, the body is the self and it is psychological, social, and interpersonal in nature. The highest Chinese virtue, *ren,* views the body-self as part of other human beings and nature (Tung, 1994).

CHAPTER 3

Self-Medication
versus Self-Soothing

THE PERCEIVED POWER OF MEDICATION

The somatization symptoms discussed in the previous chapter are generally managed with anxiolytic, antidepressant, and/or analgesic medications. Although medication is often presented as an interim or adjunctive solution, patients very quickly come to rely solely on medication and to distrust the healing resources within themselves. If anything they become increasingly fearful of their bodily sensations. Long-term reliance on medication generally works against the development of somatic awareness. Patients' strong belief in the perceived power of medication is perplexing when one considers that all mood-modifying medications rely heavily on the placebo effect, and that the placebo effect itself is a testimonial to the healing potential of inner faith. It is no accident that placebos exert some of their strongest clinical effects with chronic somatization symptoms. The problem for health professionals and patients lies in transferring the perceived origins of the placebo from the pill to the person.

Just as placebos attest directly to the power of *faith in medication,* drug dependence to a large extent reflects a *fear of not having medication.* Somatization patients who rely heavily on anxiolytic and/or analgesic medication often exhibit a tenacious belief in the continued need for the medication independent of whether the medication provides relief from their symptoms. The same dependency also exists for antidepressants, even though such drugs are considered "nonaddictive" by psychiatrists. Occurrences of placebo power and drug dependence are similar in preventing the individual from understanding and managing the condition from within.

I maintain that somatic awareness is the mind's conscious equivalent of the placebo effect. Many patients with somatic symptoms use anxiolytics even though they continue to experience symptoms. The same patients may also use hypnotic sedatives at bedtime even though they cannot sleep. Many headache sufferers consume enormous quantities of analgesic medication in spite of the fact that the medication has no impact on the intensity of their experienced pain. Migraine sufferers may use prophylactic drugs designed to prevent the onset of migraine regardless of the drugs' effectiveness on preventing the onset of migraine. When asked why they continue taking ineffective medication, patients usually reply that their symptoms would be worse without the medication. It is safer, in their eyes, to keep taking something that they know is not totally effective than to chance living with no medication at all.

The fear of having to live without medication is an extremely powerful determinant of continued use of drugs for a variety of symptoms and complaints. This fear can develop in relation to any mood-modifying medication, whether it has biological addictive properties or not. Many elderly patients never consider the possibility that they might be able to fall asleep without their regular hypnotic sedative; indeed, some individuals will actually set an alarm to awaken them at night in order to take their sleeping medication. Whether their sleep is improved is irrelevant—they believe that their medication must be swallowed and they become extremely distressed if it is not available to them taken at the suitable time. It is difficult to convince patients who are dependent on medication even to consider the possibility that they might be able to better regulate their symptoms without medication. They become nervous and even fearful when it is suggested that they no longer need medication and that they might feel better if it were removed.

Drug use behavior, once established, exhibits a life of its own, one totally independent of the actual drug effects on behavior. Drug use behavior is not easily altered and can quickly interfere with clinical efforts to develop symptom/illness control through self-regulatory somatic awareness strategies. Drug use behavior is generally incompatible with somatic awareness development: the degree of opposition increases in direct proportion to the patient's perceived need for medication. The patient who believes that he or she "must have" a particular medication for pain, anxiety, depression, or insomnia becomes distressed and frightened at the prospect of having to live without the medication. The drug has acquired "life support" status in the patient's mind and will not be readily given up.

Theoretically, there is no inherent reason why medication cannot be used in conjunction with somatic awareness to achieve symptom management. Drugs and somatic awareness can be used in a complementary, holistic fashion. Indeed, such an approach may be on the horizon since the public increasingly understands that wellness cannot be achieved with medication alone. However, the use of somatic awareness to complement medication is not yet a reality. If anything, self-medication and self-soothing stand in direct opposition to one another in the patient's mind.

Years ago, I operated a headache management program that provided patients with instruction in the use of biofeedback and relaxation training. No recommendations were made to patients regarding the present or future use of preventative and analgesic medications. I assumed that as the headache sufferers gradually gained an understanding of the psychobiological processes contributing to their headache disorder, they would gradually reduce their reliance on medication. I was surprised to discover that although some patients exhibited this pattern, the majority did not. Over the years, many of the patients who clearly benefited from biobehavioral intervention nevertheless resumed full use of medication or started new medication for controlling their headache pain. It came as a surprise to me that these headache sufferers, in spite of exposure to multiple sessions of relaxation training and biofeedback, often had very little understanding of how to manage their symptoms without medication. In conversation, they mentioned the benefits of therapy but they seemed much more enthusiastic about the latest migraine medication they were trying. It was evident that these patients had not learned to trust their own internal experiences for managing their headaches. A contributing reason for this failure may have been the unaltered use of medication during the biobehavioral training sessions. Their faith in medication, even ineffective medication, was far greater than their faith in themselves.

Why patients feel that they must rely on something other than themselves or believe that they "desperately" need an anxiolytic or analgesic medication is a complicated issue. The fact that people often prefer mood-altering and analgesic drugs may simply mean that they do not know what else to do since no one has made the effort to show them how to manage without medication. Self-control of symptoms has not had a very long history in health care. Until recently, occurrences of symptom recovery in the absence of medicine were often dismissed as "just a placebo effect"—the implication was that the patient was not

really sick in the first place. This view is changing: it is now recognized
that the psychobiological processes that mediate the placebo effect
have the potential to bring about a revolution in the way illness is managed.

THE PLACEBO IN TRANSITION

Placebos have always had a soothing connotation. Discussions of
placebo phenomena, for example, generally begin with the original
Latin meaning of the term which is "I shall please." Traditionally placebo medication is prescribed to please or soothe the patient rather
than to serve a therapeutic purpose. At the clinical level, a "placebo" is
defined as an intervention designed to simulate medical therapy, even
though the clinician believes that it has no utility for the presenting
condition. According to this view, the *soothing* nature of the placebo is
more important for the patient than its medical value. The main point
of this chapter is that such soothing does have great medical value if
properly understood. The healing process evoked by placebo is real,
occurs through psychobiological processes within the person, and has
potential for being consciously controlled through somatic awareness.
    The history of the placebo effect can be characterized as the his-
tory of the human need to swallow something. All kinds of strange
ingredients have been willingly ingested throughout the ages to cure
disease. Ground-up mummy (of the Egyptian variety), crocodile dung,
soles of old shoes, and mice have all been recommended at one time or
another. Each of these swallowed substances must have "worked" for
some individuals at least some of the time. The practice of swallowing
unusual substances to maintain or restore health continues. A newspa-
per report described hundreds of scientists meeting in India for the
first World Conference on Auto-Urine Therapy. Drinking one's own
urine is a 5,000-year-old therapy for diseases ranging from heart disease to cancer. The "Water of Life" treatment requires consumption of
one or two glasses of fresh urine a day in conjunction with regular
body massages using stale urine at least 4 days old.
    Shapiro and Morris (1978) defined "placebo" as "any therapy or
component of therapy that is deliberately used for its non-specific, psychological or psychophysiological effect, or that is used for its presumed specific effect, but is without specific activity for the condition
being treated" (p. 371). The definition of placebo as nonspecific in
nature and without specific activity had the unintended effect of reinforcing a view of the placebo as unreal, unwanted, and more representative of quackery than of "true" treatment effects (Wall, 1992). The

zeitgeist surrounding this definition also created a sense of embarrassment rather than accomplishment in those individuals who responded
positively in the presence of a placebo. Until recently, improvement in
response to placebo administration was not viewed as indicative of the
potential healing powers within the individual but more as a sign that
the individual was not sick in the first place.

Grünbaum (1993) attempted to resolve the distinction between
"specific" and "nonspecific" elements of therapy with the proposal that
the terms specific and nonspecific effects be replaced with "characteristic" versus "incidental" components of any particular drug or other
treatment method. A therapeutic theory that advocates the use of a
certain treatment demands the inclusion of certain characteristic constituents; any treatment process will, however, also have certain other
constituents that are incidental relative to the therapeutic theory. A
treatment variable, according to Grünbaum, is a placebo when its therapeutic effect is not due to its characteristic components but to some
of its incidental components. This redefinition of specific and nonspecific effects avoids the issue of the origins of the placebo effect. It
implies that the incidental effects reside within the therapy rather than
the person and further implies that their nature will eventually be identified and incorporated into the characteristic treatment process. But
Grünbaum's model ignores the fact that the source of placebo power
lies within the person.

Placebo Research in Review

When placebos are used in research, experimenter bias and patient
expectancy are reduced by using a double blind-procedure in which neither the treatment administrator nor the patient is aware of which treatment is being administered to which patient. The randomized double-
blind control trial is considered the "gold standard" of the pharmaceutical industry. The preferred design procedure is a 2 × 2 factorial design
known as the *balanced placebo design*. In this design, half of the subjects
are told that they will be receiving the drug, while the other half are told
that they will not receive the drug. But in *each* of these groups, half of the
subjects actually receive the drug, while the other half do not. Thus the
design consists of four groups in which subjects (1) are told that they are
being given a drug and *do* receive the drug; (2) are told that they will be
given a drug and *do not* receive the drug; (3) are told that they will not be
given a drug and *do* receive the drug; and (4) are told that they will not be
given a drug and *do not* receive the drug.

It is often stated that placebos are effective with 35% of people.

This view can be traced to a classic study by Beecher (1955). Beecher reviewed 15 double-blind studies containing 1,082 patients and observed an average 35% placebo response rate. Beecher's review included studies of postsurgical pain, angina, headache, nausea, drug-induced mood changes, cough, anxiety and tension, and the common cold. It is now recognized that the 35% figure grossly underestimates the true power of placebo effects. Even in the Beecher paper, there was large variability in reported placebo responsiveness, with a range of 15% to 58% of patients reporting satisfactory relief.

Roberts and colleagues (Roberts, Kewman, Mercier, & Hovell, 1993) proposed that the power of placebo effects is much greater in naturalistic settings, and that in some cases may reach values as high as 100%. They maintain that double-blind study designs, like those utilized in the Beecher review, rule out the optimism, conviction, and persuasive abilities of the therapist that occur under normal clinical circumstances. Thus reports of the power of placebos based upon double-blind studies seriously underestimate the real power of placebos.

To examine the possibility that placebo effects are greater when both the patient and the physician believe in the efficacy of the treatment, Roberts et al. reviewed the treatment effectiveness initially reported as supportive of several pharmacological and surgical treatments but later reported to be ineffective. The clinical trials were initially "open" and not subject to blind experimental procedures. They identified five such treatments:

1. *Glomectomy.* This surgical treatment was used in the 1960s to treat asthma. The treatment involved separating the carotid body or glomus from the adventitial mass of the external carotid artery in order to correct a presumed reflex disturbance thought to be responsible for asthma. Over 6,000 asthma sufferers were treated in the absence of controlled clinical trials before the procedure was found to be useless and discontinued.

2. *Levamisole treatment of herpes simplex virus.* Levamisole is a immunomodulating drug that showed great promise, presumably because of its ability to enhance cell-mediated immunity. Double-blind studies failed to find support for the treatment.

3. *Photodynamic activation for treating herpes simplex virus.* This treatment was advocated for herpes in the early 1970s but abandoned late in the same decade. The treatment involved rupturing the herpes lesion and painting the region with a dye, and then exposing it to fluorescent light. The combination of dye and light was presumed to inactivate the virus. Of 169 patients treated in uncontrolled trials, 89% showed good to

excellent outcomes. Double-blind studies again showed, however, no differences between treatment and control groups.

   4. *Organic solvent treatment for herpes.* This treatment was initially reported to have 100% success but was quickly discontinued as useless.

   5. *Gastric freezing for ulcers.* The stomach lining was frozen in order to suppress gastric secretions. The technique had good success initially but later failed to have therapeutic value.

A summary of the initial results for these five treatments based on uncontrolled clinical trials are presented in Table 3.1. The average reported effectiveness of these treatments was 40.2% excellent results, 29.6% good results, and 30.3% poor results—which, according to Roberts et al. (1993), results in an average total of 70% positive outcomes, twice the percentage reported by Beecher (1955). Roberts et al. used these data to argue that placebo effects are extremely powerful when both patients and doctors strongly believe in the anticipated treatment effectiveness.

An unexplained phenomenon illustrating the subtle nature of placebo effects is the observation that drug-produced response profiles and placebo-produced response profiles across different drugs seem to parallel one another. In a review of 11 double-blind studies of clinical pain, Evans (1974) found that the effectiveness of a placebo seemed to be directly proportional to the perceived efficacy of the drug that the doctor and the patient believed they were using. The more powerful the drug administered, the more powerful the placebo response observed. The placebo was found to be 54% as effective as aspirin (a mild analgesic), 56% as effective as Darvon (a somewhat stronger analgesic), and 56% as effective as morphine (a much stronger analgesic).

TABLE 3.1. Reported Outcomes in Clinical Trials of Five Ineffective Treatments

Treatment	Sample size	Reported outcomes (%)		
		Excellent	Good	Poor
Glomectomy	5,976	41.0	30.2	28.8
Levamisole	139	48.2	36.7	15.1
Photodynamic activation	169	59.2	30.2	10.6
Organic solvents	49	38.7	32.7	28.6
Gastric freezing	598	24.5	20.3	55.2
Combined data	6,931	40.2	29.6	30.3

These observations indicate that the "pharmacological" properties of the placebo tend to closely mimic the pharmacological properties of the active drug with which it is being compared.

Fine, Roberts, Gillette, and Child (1994) observed a similar parallel response profile of placebo and active drug profiles in a study of phentolamine injections for the control of chronic back pain. Phentolamine is an alpha-adrenergic antagonist that blocks sympathetic nervous system activity. The subjects were told that they would receive six separate infusions during two separate sessions separated by a week, and that different concentrations of the active drug, including no active drug at all, would be given in a random order that was unknown to the investigator. In one session the subject received placebo-only infusions and in the other session the subject received a single injection of phentolamine in injection number 3 or 5. Each session was 2 hours in length, with an infusion of phentolamine or placebo occurring every 15 minutes. Subjects rated their back pain at the end of each 15-minute period and also gave a rating to a stimulus-evoked cold pain elicited by application of an alcohol pad followed by drying. The response profiles across the two sessions to phentolamine and placebo only were quite similar for some subjects. If it took time for a subject to exhibit analgesia to the phentolamine, it also required a similar amount of time for the subject to develop analgesia to the placebo. Thus, a slowly developing placebo response mimicked the slowly developing phentolamine response. One patient reported in a telephone interview after the placebo-only session complete absence of pain for 8 hours, which was her first experience without pain for years. Unfortunately, the pain returned after the brief period of complete relief.

Sapirstein and Kirsch (1996) completed an elaborate meta-analysis of the placebo effect of antidepressant medications. They calculated response rates for over 3,000 patients who had received antidepressant medication, placebo, psychotherapy, or no treatment in 39 studies. In presenting their study, they adopted a distinction between the response to and the effect of treatments. A response to a drug is not necessarily the same as a drug effect. Drug responses may occur as a function of nonspecific factors, with the drug itself having very little effect. In their meta-analysis, they defined "response" as any alteration in behavior or condition following a treatment; they defined "effect" as a change that is significantly greater than the change observed in an appropriate control group. Thus, drug effect was defined as the difference between the drug response and the placebo response, while the placebo effect was defined as the difference between the placebo response and the response to no treatment or the passage of time (studies show that approximately 50% of depressed patients improve with the passage of time alone). Following the analyses, the study claimed to have found that 27% of the response to antidepressant medication is a true pharmacological effect, 50% is due to the psychological impact of administering the medication, and 23% is due to additional nonspecific factors. The results of the study indicate that close to 75% of the response to drugs is not related to the pharmacological qualities of the antidepressant medication.

There is a growing consensus that it is time to develop a new understanding of the psychobiological phenomena associated with the placebo effect. Rather than leave the placebo effect to nonspecific, subconscious, and nondeliberative processes, there is recognition of the need to experience the placebo as a specific healing force within the active conscious mind. Placebo explanations based on anxiety reduction and cognitive expectancy state that placebos obtain their healing power because of pervasive cultural beliefs associated with sickness and health. Beliefs that one has a serious illness can lead to feelings of depression and anxiety; conversely, beliefs in the curative power of modern medicine counteract such feelings of depression and anxiety. If a person really believes that "this medicine is going to cure me," the new belief will be incompatible with holding on to sickness beliefs. The placebo belief will produce emotional responses of hope and calm that are antagonistic to depression and anxiety. Lundh (1987) suggested that the more a person's illness involves psychological components of anxiety and depression, the more susceptible he/she will be to the induction of placebo effects. Moreover, a positive cycle may be produced, whereby positive placebo beliefs will make the person selectively attentive to any signs of improved health.

Lundh's psychological analysis of the placebo is similar to explanations that invoke faith as the crucial psychological construct. A person is said to have faith in something when he or she has absolutely no doubt about it. A person who has faith in a procedure does not question whether that procedure will work he or she simply assumes that it will work. Moreover, patients who have faith in a treatment will begin to behave as persons who have been cured. If they have complete faith in the treatment, they see themselves as being in the process of being cured, and therefore behave like persons who are cured. Faith in a treatment, then, extends beyond simply having positive expectancies, conviction, or hope:

> If an individual does not merely expect to be cured, but takes it for granted that he or she *has* been cured or is well on the road to a cure, then that individual is less likely to see things as evidence to the contrary,

and accordingly, is more likely to act in a manner consistent with and facilitative of cure.

. . . Consider a man who suffers from chronic muscle contraction headaches. If he is given a prescription of placebo pills, and if he has faith in the efficacy of the putative medicine, he will take it for granted that his headache problem has been cured and will treat himself accordingly. He may no longer expect to be stricken with headaches; he may cease to worry about being regularly incapacitated; he may experience a lifting of a tremendous burden, and may perhaps celebrate by spending his newly "won" time in pursuing various pleasurable and relaxing endeavors for which he previously felt ineligible; and he may no longer present himself to others (or to himself) as a headache sufferer. (Plotkin, 1985, pp. 241–242)

But psychological explanations of the placebo based on expectancy or faith are usually in the minds of others, not in the mind of the person responding to the placebo (Plotkin, 1985). The person exhibiting a placebo response in the presence of a sugar pill does not understand that his/her therapeutic change is the result of inner actions related to faith, expectancy, and other variables. If the patient recognized that the improvement is due to placebo, then the improvement would not be attributed to the placebo but to some inner self-regulatory process. The question remains whether it is possible to shift the source of placebo power to the individual and still achieve the same therapeutic effectiveness.

Directing individuals to trust their inner experience will take reeducation and appreciation of the power within the person. Current discussions of the placebo are shifting in their emphasis from outer variables that initiate the placebo effect to process variables within the person. One current definition, for example, emphasizes the central nervous system (CNS) processes in defining "placebo" as *a response initiated in the cortex, whence neural, endocrine, and immune influences emerge to set in motion a beneficial action at the molecular level* (Gordon, 1996, p. 119). Of course, this definition begs the question of the nature of the mental process that initiates the cortical response.

It makes practical sense to understand the otherwise mysterious placebo in terms of somatic awareness. By being aware of bodily sensations that accompany treatments known to be associated with a placebo effect, individuals can learn to initiate similar and possibly more sustained changes without necessarily swallowing a pill or having their body regularly purged of impurities. Such an explanation of placebo phenomena remains a hypothesis; if supported it will have enormous influence on how we interpret the operation of all drugs and therapies.

The hypothesis suggesting that somatic awareness be used to reconceptualize the placebo effect receives support from critiques of the double-blind methodology. The double-blind design assumes that it is possible to separate the psychological and the physiological effects associated with taking a drug. The effect of taking a drug consists of two components: a specific physiological component and a nonspecific psychological component. The effect of a placebo, on the other hand, is assumed to consist of only one component: a nonspecific psychological component. Researchers assume that in using a placebo–control group design that it possible to numerically isolate the improvement rate due to psychological factors from the improvement rate due to physiological factors. The placebo design assumes, however, that the psychological and physiological effects of using medication are independent and can be examined in an additive fashion without having to consider the interactive or psychobiological nature of response to drugs. However, there are many examples that suggest that it is the interaction between psychological and biological variables that is crucial in determining positive response to drugs.

The double-blind condition is now recognized, at least with some medications, as not necessarily being "blind" to the participants involved. A study cited by Fisher and Greenberg (1989) asked physicians and patients being treated for depression to guess at the end of 6 weeks of treatment whether they had received an active drug treatment or a placebo. Both patients and physicians were able to correctly guess the appropriate conditions at high levels of accuracy (79% and 87%). Also of importance is the finding that a patient's ability to correctly guess whether treatment was placebo or active drug was predictive of treatment success. When the patients were grouped into those who had or who had not responded to the treatments, it was found that responders were more accurate than nonresponders in identifying whether they had received an active drug or a placebo (Fisher & Greenberg, 1989).

Greenberg and Fisher (1989) proposed that the vital source of information with therapeutic potential within the double-blind design are the cues supplied by the *bodily sensations* activated by the drug. These bodily sensations, it is important to understand, are considered distinct from the CNS changes that are believed to be responsible for observed improvements. The tricyclic antidepressants (TCAs), for example, are believed to block neuronal reuptake of serotonin within the CNS. The use of these drugs is also associated with a number of troublesome bodily side effects which include tremor, dry mouth, sweating, and constipation. Inert placebos might initiate some bodily sensations but nothing of the magnitude of an active TCA. Subjects in a drug trial are generally warned to expect certain side effects; if they do not experience them, they may conclude that they have been given a placebo, or that the drug is ineffective for them. Conversely, those who do experience side effects may feel that the drug is working and will not think that they have received inert or ineffective medication.

Greenberg and Fisher (1989) described a review by Thomson (1982) of a large number of double-blind placebo-controlled studies of TCAs. Thomson discovered that of those that used an inert placebo, 59% found a superior therapeutic effect for the TCA. Of those that used an active placebo, atropine, only 14% of the studies reviewed showed a superior effect for TCAs. Atropine produces anticholinergic symptoms similar to those associated with use of TCAs, and in this respect would function as an active placebo by arousing body sensations that affirm a therapeutic agent had been ingested. The notion that body responses have therapeutic significance would apply to both active placebos and drugs. An active drug may not only be more easily recognized as a "real" treatment but may also stimulate special somatic awareness feelings that can influence various levels of behavior.

The new selective serotonin reuptake inhibitor (SSRI) antidepressants, such as fluoxetine (Prozac), were initially considered to be relatively free of side effects. If this were true, then any therapeutic effect associated with these drugs could not be explained in terms of patient awareness of bodily feelings associated with side effects. Greenberg and colleagues (Greenberg, Bornstein, Zborowski, Fisher, & Greenberg, 1994), however, argue that a proportion of the antidepressant activity associated with fluoxetine might follow the same model as outlined for the TCAs. The SSRIs are now recognized to be associated with their own distinctive side effects which include nausea, nervousness, and insomnia. Greenberg et al. examined 13 double-blind studies of fluoxetine and found that the overall improvement rate was similar to what has been reported for other types of antidepressants. Although they were unable to find studies that had used an active placebo, they did observe a positive correlation between the number of patients who reported side effects and outcome ratings: the greater the number of patients in a study with reported side effects, the better the outcome ratings became.

Moving placebo processes from external sources to internal attributes will require changes in the way we understand illness and its management. I recall a patient with multiple chronic pain problems that she attributed to an advancing but unknown disease. Numerous negative neurological investigations could not dissuade her from this belief. She experienced severe migraines and tried various medications to control the pain. Although not drug-dependent, she could not accept the idea that she might be able, through increased awareness of observable tension in her neck, shoulders, and face, to reduce the frequency of her headache episodes. She struggled with trying to become more somatically aware, but established beliefs and habits are slow to change. One day, while standing on a table to change a light bulb, she fell and struck her head. For 3 weeks, while her head healed, she experienced no episodes of migraine pain. However, once the injury healed, the migraines returned to their preinjury level of severity. She could not understand why her headaches disappeared during the period of convalescence from the fall. It is likely that during the healing period, her habitual psychobiological response patterns were altered, leading to less general bodily distress and temporary migraine relief. Unfortunately, she could not make these connections within her somatic self. When the headaches returned, her physician decided to try a vitamin B_{12} injection. Once again the headaches completely disappeared, only to return after several injections. This example demonstrates the need for and power of faith in an external treatment. Accessing this healing power in oneself requires placing trust in one's own embodiment.

Transitional Relatedness

A multitude of psychological and situational variables contribute to the placebo effect, but only one variable is directly relevant to somatic awareness. Humans may have an inner need for soothing. The existence of such a need is best described in psychoanalytic theory. Psychoanalytic writers speak on the one hand of a need for inner soothing and on the other hand of an inhibition against self-soothing or taking care of oneself. Soothing is necessary, but its source is often reserved for agents outside of oneself. In strict psychoanalytic theory, carrying out any form of "mothering," or soothing activities, is reserved for one's external mother and is forbidden to the child and, in later life, to the adult as well unless these mothering functions are successfully internalized during the formative years (Krystal, 1982).

The inability to self-soothe has its origins in the concept of *transitional relatedness,* first proposed by Winnicott (1953). Winnicott viewed transitional relatedness as an experiential state comprised of both inner and outer reality—a kind of intermediate state of consciousness. He expressed the view that children and adults have a universal need for soothing relationships and soothing objects. The popularity of the teddy bear with both children and adults represents a familiar example of a soothing transitional object. The attachment of the cartoon character Linus to his blanket is another familiar example of certain objects acquiring self-soothing power. Prior to Winnicott's article, the comforting value of the teddy bear and otherwise worthless objects had not drawn scholarly attention. Today the transitional object is regarded as symbolic of developmental processes of self-nurturance or self-soothing within the individual.

Transitional relatedness is different from other forms of emotional relatedness. It is a unique experience between the individual and the object. Horton (1981) defined "transitional relatedness" as "the person's unique experience of an object, whether animate or inanimate, tangible or intangible, in a reliably soothing manner based on the object's associative or symbolic connection with an abiding, mainly maternal primary process presence" (p. 34). In day-to-day life, any object, real or symbolic, can be used to create a soothing sensation. It is entirely reasonable to seek out objects to facilitate the somatic awareness process. The child (or adult) with a teddy bear knows that the teddy bear is nothing but cloth and stuffing but for the moment objective reality is suspended in favor of attributing to the bear the feelings that he needs to experience at the moment. Soothing experiences involving the teddy bear, blanket, or some other soft item become interwoven with the internal life of the owner.

According to Horton (1981), the child's need for self-soothing evolves into the adult's need for solace. He prefers the word "solace" to get away from what he sees as childish connotations associated with the word "soothing" and to give this state the broadest meaning possible, from hugging a teddy bear to engaging in spiritual activities. Over time, external objects become less important in achieving solace, while symbolic experiences become more important. Thus, for an adult, taking a walk or listening to specific music can create a sense of solace. Each individual has his or her way of relating to the soothing archetype of the *paradisal mother*. Horton (1988) provided an example of how fishermen in the darkness of the stormy Atlantic would experience a shared vision of an old woman sitting in the bow of their boat singing lullabies to them. She was known as the "cradle woman," the old nurse who would rock them to sleep when they were small. Many adults, unfortunately, have not developed or have misplaced this fundamental human healing ability.

There is a striking similarity between the soothing nature of transitional objects and the soothing nature of medication. Individuals who rely on medication to sleep, to settle themselves, or to reduce pain can become frantic if the medication is not at hand. Once the pill is ingested, however, the individuals experience an immediate release and comfort, often prior to the dissolving of the capsule in their stomach. This is not a trivial phenomenon; indeed, it may well contribute in a significant manner to a drug's overall effectiveness. The ritualistic act of swallowing medication, whatever its chemical content, seems to alleviate patient fears and insecurities associated with having "to go it alone." It may even explain, at least in part, the healing effect of chicken soup when we are ill.

The universal need for transitional objects is not open to question. But can people be just as effective in caring for themselves when the need arises? Can people self-soothe with the same clinical effectiveness through somatic awareness? Or is it better to use their favorite transitional object to maximize their ability to self-soothe? The thesis of this book is that people need not rely on drugs as transitional objects: there are better ways to achieve similar benefits through their own somatic experiences.

A holistic view of placebo processes is needed to capture the psychobiological and experiential nature as well as the self-governing potential of placebo phenomena. Although faith in drugs, physicians, religion, and a variety of other "transitional" interventions is important, individuals need to be able to experience the healing processes within themselves, to know, in effect, if their conscious strategies are initiating the desired bodily changes within themselves. We are, in effect, shifting the healing processes that are part of the placebo effect to somatic awareness. Somatic awareness represents the systematic and unifying experiential equivalent of the placebo effect.

The promotion of somatic awareness as an alternative to placebos logically calls for the elimination of placebo use in clinical practice. If health professionals are truly interested in identifying the inseparable healing nature of the mind–body experience and developing patient partnerships based on mutual respect and trust, then it is inconceivable to advocate a strategy that involves the deliberate use of deceit to help patients. There are medical practitioners who believe placebos continue to have an important place in medicine, especially in the treatment of anxiety, depression, and pain. With depression, for example, claims are made that successful outcomes using placebos are close to active agents (50% in both cases) and that the placebo has the advantage of having no side effects. But I believe that placebos should not be used under any circumstances.

Fortunately, the use of placebos and deception in research and clinical practice is likely to decrease, if not disappear. The ethics of giving placebos, both for therapeutics and for controlled research, has become, in the words of Gordon (1996), "a minefield of legal, social, philosophical and religious hazards inviting continued study by the ethics committee and other professionals from lay and academic fields" (p. 124). Patient rights movements have challenged the notion of the physician having absolute control. In research, there have been calls to abandon the use of the placebo design in conditions where there are known effective treatments. The argument is that randomization of a subject to placebo treatment when an established effective treatment is available unnecessarily exposes the subject to further harm. In clinical practice the use of placebos is challenged on the grounds that deception risks loss of confidence in the physician and generates a distorted view of drugs. One counterargument is that the physician prescribing the placebo might tell the patient that the pill is a placebo known to be effective in treating the symptom. In this manner, a clinician prescribing a pill placebo to a patient would not be lying. It is doubtful, however, that the placebo would be effective under such an administration. Placebos have no place in modern health care because the public no longer wants to be deceived. Partnerships between patients and professionals need to be based on mutual respect and trust, not on deception.

THE HOLISTIC NATURE OF DRUG DEPENDENCE

Presenting somatic awareness as an alternative to the placebo is meant to demonstrate the potential inner healing power that is available to the individual. Harnessing this healing power in clinical practice is another matter. Most individuals who are using anxiolytic, analgesic, and (to a lesser extent) antidepressant medication to control somatic symptoms are dependent on the medication. I mentioned in the opening section of this chapter that patients have very strong beliefs that their medications are absolutely necessary to maintain their health. They have a difficult time understanding that it is possible for bodily awareness and medication to work synergistically or comprehending that they might be able to achieve the same bodily control without medication. It is as if medication magically frees them from having to make any changes within themselves in order to manage their symptoms.

The pharmaceutical industry claims that by using the appropriate medication, the individual will gain the freedom to live life without further difficulty with anxiety, pain, insomnia, and so forth. Drug use, however, is never a passive process: it is accompanied by dynamic changes in the individual's psychobiological makeup. The phrase "drugs can help a whole bunch, but there is no free lunch" (Rosenthal, 1993, p. 439) emphasizes that drugs should be avoided when possible, mainly because of unwanted side effects and the risk of abuse. But the potential difficulties of drug use go beyond the experience of unwanted symptoms and occasional abuse. At the symptom level, drug use can very quickly create a paradoxical situation in which the use of the drug leads to a worsening of the very symptoms the drug is designed to control. The frequency and strength of these drug-dependent symptoms is widely underestimated both by the physicians who prescribe the medication and by the patients who ingest it.

Medical specialists used to try to separate the physical and psychological dimensions of drug dependence. Although some clinicians still speak as if the distinction exists, there is a growing appreciation of the psychobiological nature of all forms of drug dependence. Efforts to separate psychological and physical dependence are no longer considered appropriate for understanding the drug-dependent individual. This is just as true of the street addict as of the medical patient. In trying to appreciate the experiential state of these individuals, it is advantageous to view drug dependence as characterized by an overwhelming belief in the need for medication and accompanying fears of not being able to survive without medication.

"Physical dependence" is defined as an altered state of biology, such that when the drug is withdrawn a set of biological events are initiated that are distinct from the events that would occur with normal function (Jaffe, 1992). Physical dependence is "a physiological phenomenon solely defined by the development of an abstinence syndrome following abrupt discontinuation of therapy, substantial dose reduction or administration of an antagonist drug" (Portenoy, 1996, p. 22). The determinants of physical dependence are viewed entirely in biological terms and include concepts such as biological half-life and mode of metabolism. Physical dependence can develop within a single cell, a complex of cells, or the whole organism. The initial signs of physical dependence can occur as soon as the drug receptors are activated. A single dose of benzodiazepine or opioid, for example, can initiate evidence of developing dependence as discontinuation of these drugs may lead to minor physical symptoms such as yawning, nausea, and sweating.

The best clinical description of drug dependence is a syndrome in which the use of a drug is given a much higher priority than other behaviors that once had higher value (Jaffe, 1992). The existence of drug dependence varies along a psychobiological (rather than a purely physiological) continuum. The term "addiction" refers to severe instances of dependence. Addiction is characterized "as a psychological and behavioral syndrome in which there is drug craving, compulsive use and other aberrant drug-related behaviors, and relapse after withdrawal" (Portenoy & Payne, 1992, p. 692). This definition of addiction was developed by experts who had the street addict in mind rather than the medical patient. The term "drug-dependent" is more suitable for the medical patient.

The recognition of the psychobiological nature of drug dependence is evident in the appreciation of commonalities across drug-dependent behaviors. Patients who become dependent on one medication tend to become dependent on other medications. Thus, the patient who is dependent on morphine or codeine for pain control is often dependent on benzodiazepine for anxiety, a hypnotic sedative for sleep, and possibly an antidepressant for depression. Because of gastro-intestinal effects, the patient may also be dependent on several medications for nausea and constipation or diarrhea. All these medications might, to some extent, be mediated by common psychobiological processes and contribute to the same drug-dependency syndrome. The drug management of such patients is extremely difficult because withdrawal of one drug will not solve the problem nor will efforts to replace the "addictive" medications with ones that are pharmacologically "less addictive."

The important commonalities across drug-dependent behaviors (Donovan, 1988) that must be recognized and monitored include the following:

1. The drug experience represents a powerful and immediate technique for changing one's mood and body sensations.
2. Changes in arousal associated with pain, distress, or negative moods (e.g., depression, boredom, loneliness) tend to increase the likelihood of needing any available drug.
3. The living environment is a powerful determinant of the need for medication.
4. The drug-dependent experience is generally considered beyond the individual's control.
5. Relapse following efforts to discontinue drug use is very common and is under the control of individual, situational, and physiological factors.
6. Drug dependence is not inherently related to a given drug; thus substitution of one drug for another drug may lead to a relapse in the use of the first drug and/or dependence on the second drug. It is the person who becomes drug-dependent, and this dependency is often associated with a number of drugs.
7. It is possible, usually with professional assistance, to overcome drug dependency.

Many physicians believe that there is too much concern and scare-mongering regarding the dangers of drug dependency.

Portenoy (1996), for example, in trying to minimize growing fears surrounding the clinical use of opioids for controlling chronic pain, proposes a distinction between drug-seeking behaviors that are *probably predictive* of addiction and drug-seeking behaviors that are *less predictive* of addiction. He lists the following behaviors as *probably predictive* of addiction: selling prescription drugs, injecting oral formulations, obtaining prescription drugs from nonmedical sources, multiple episodes of prescription "loss," and current abuse of illicit drugs. Very few, if any, patients seen in general medical practice would meet such a demanding definition of addiction or drug dependency. They would, however, readily meet his definition of drug behaviors that are *less predictive* of addiction. These behaviors include aggressive complaining about the need for more drug, drug hoarding during periods of reduced symptoms, requesting specific drugs, openly acquiring similar drugs from other medical sources, unsanctioned dose escalation or other noncompliance with therapy on one or two occasions, unapproved use of drug to treat another symptom, and resistance to change in therapy because of fear of a return of severe symptoms.

Portenoy argues that we should be willing to tolerate considerable drug-seeking behavior in patients before calling it addictive or drug-dependent. In his view, the drug-seeking actions of medical patients are instances of *therapeutic dependence* rather than of drug dependence or addiction. Complaining about the need for more drugs or increasing the dosage without consultation is simply evidence of the patient's belief that medication is required in the same way that a diabetic patient without access to insulin may seek out insulin or an angina patient may seek out nitrate—in other words, the drugs are needed for an appropriate therapeutic outcome, not for a "fix." This position turns a blind eye to the countless patients who, although not stealing opioids or free-basing, are exhibiting major withdrawal symptoms and in whom drug-seeking behaviors, although occurring within the confines of the health care system, cause enormous difficulties with their treatment. Furthermore, unless a substantial number of the behaviors listed as "less predictive of addiction" are controlled or changed, it remains virtually impossible to provide these individuals with a significant degree of symptom control through somatic awareness training or any other therapy.

Psychoanalytic writers have long recognized that mood drugs are used to control more than surface symptoms. They can also be used as a defense against psychological suffering and self-regulatory deficiencies (Brehm & Khantzian, 1992). Drug-dependent individuals describe their use of an anxiolytic or analgesic substance not only in terms of specific symptom management, but also in terms of a need to maintain a sense of inner equilibrium or homeostasis. Specific symptoms may not even be mentioned. They might describe using on analgesic not because of a specific pain but rather because of "pain all over" or to feel "better," "okay," "not overwhelmed," or "not out of control." This state is often described in terms of a need to maintain a psychological or emotional equilibrium on the part of the individual—a need to avoid psychological suffering. Although the negative emotional state may vary from pain to depression to anxiety, the individual feels a collective need to use medication to avoid the suffering that accompanies all these states.

> Recently, more emphasis has been placed on understanding addiction as "self-medication" to alleviate suffering, with less emphasis on severe psychopathology. For example, pain-relieving properties of the opiates help the user modulate disturbing, rageful feelings that are the source of much suffering in their lives, often originating in past experiences in which they were victims, perpetrators, or both. The sedative-hypnotics can help tense, emotionally restricted individuals to experience walled-off affect and to overcome related fears concerning human closeness, dependency, and intimacy. . . .
>
> Substance abusers adopt the use of drugs as a means to control feelings of helplessness and rage. . . . By acting to take control of one's own affective state, addictive behavior may serve to restore a sense of control when there is a perception that control or power has been lost or taken away. (Brehm & Khantzian, 1992, p. 109)

Somatic awareness remains the core of therapeutic focus in guiding patients to manage the multitude of emotions and interpersonal situations that exacerbate their symptoms and need for medication. Patients who are using drugs to prevent themselves from "feeling bad" or "being unable to go on" also experience a multitude of somatic symptoms that at times are barely mentioned in clinical sessions. It is good practice during sessions to gently direct these individuals toward these neglected bodily experiences. Stomach distress, chest pain, headache, labored breathing, and/or throat tightness are symptoms that are readily identifiable by these patients and that can be used as a focus of intervention. By proceeding in this fashion, the patient is able to gain a degree of control over the frightening sensations that accompany these symptoms and, with a clearer mind, begin working on the psychological and interpersonal issues that may be exacerbating these symptoms and the need for medication.

ANXIETY AND THE BENZODIAZEPINES

The benzodiazepines are by far the most frequently used class of drugs in medical practice for anxiety-related conditions. The benzodiazepines are generally described as highly effective for treating anxiety disorders. Less often mentioned is their very significant potential for abuse and chemical dependency. Studies have shown that between 70% and 90% of patients receiving a clinical trial of benzodiazepines for panic anxiety experience a return and worsening of their symptoms following discontinuation of the drug. The anxiety symptoms that return are often more severe than pretreatment symptom levels (Otto, Pollack, Meltzer-Brody, & Rosenbaum, 1992). This paradoxical drug effect on symptoms may remain undetected and may negatively impact the patient for the duration of his/her life. This pattern of drug withdrawal followed by symptom worsening and increased drug use represents an enormous cost to the patient, the patient's family, and the health care system.

Numerous benzodiazepines are available. They are variously described as "anxiolytics," "sedatives," "muscle relaxants," "intravenous anesthetics," and "anticonvulsants." Although certain benzodiazepines are singled out as specific for each of these uses, they are all similarly effective in the short-term management of anxiety. The benzodiazepines differ from each other primarily in terms of their biological half-lives and whether their metabolism is associated with the presence of active metabolites (Julien, 1995). The biological half-life of a drug is the time required for the drug concentration in the blood to fall by one-half. It is the time required for the body to eliminate the drug through metabolism (by the liver) and the excretion of metabolites (by the kidneys).

Some drug half-lives can be measured in hours, some in days, and some in weeks. Diazepam (Valium) is classified as a long-acting benzodiazepine with an elimination half-life of 24 hours (range = 20–50 hours) . During metabolism diazepam is also biotransformed into the long-acting active metabolite nordiazepam with a half-life of 60 hours (range = 50–100 hours). Lorazepam (Ativan) is an intermediate-acting benzodiazepine with a half-life of 15 hours (range = 10–24 hours). Alprazolam (Xanax), oxazepam (Serax), and triazolam (Halcion) are examples of short-acting benzodiazepines with half-lives ranging from 12 hours for alprazolam, to 8 hours for oxazepam, and to 2.5 hours for triazolam. A shorter half-life is deemed of value in treating insomnia, as the morning "cloudiness" with a longer acting benzodiazepine is avoided. Unfortunately, the same short half-life can result in a rapid drop in serum level, resulting in a high incidence of withdrawal reactions characterized by nocturnal panic and rebound insomnia.

There is drug accumulation in the blood with repeated drug use. Usually an individual takes a repeat dose before the previous dose is fully cleared from the body; as a result, the drug builds up in the body. It can often take five to six half-lives to eliminate a drug completely from the body. The elderly have a compromised ability to metabolize long-acting benzodiazepines and their metabolites. The elimination half-life in the elderly for the drug and its active metabolite can often be more than 10 days. Since it takes about six half-lives to rid the body of a drug, it may thus require 60 days for the body of an elderly patient to become free of diazepam, even after a single dose. Elderly patients can readily become cognitively confused from the prolonged use of a long-acting benzodiazepine such as diazepam.

The concept of the benzodiazepine receptor combined with the amino acid transmitter gamma-aminobutyric acid (GABA) is at the heart of understanding the action of benzodiazepine drugs. GABA is the most prevalent inhibitory transmitter in the CNS; it is believed to be present in 30% of brain synapses. GABA is also known to have excitatory effects at some synapses. Brain benzodiazepine receptors are found in diverse regions throughout the forebrain and the brainstem, with the most dense regions including the olfactory bulbs, hippocampus, amygdala, cerebellum, and lamina IV of the cortex. There are two different types of GABA receptors, $GABA_a$ and $GABA_b$. The $GABA_a$ receptor, when occupied by GABA, leads to an increased flow of negative chloride ions through chloride channels into the cell, thereby hyperpolarizing the cell and inhibiting its function. $GABA_b$ receptors operate as neuromodulators and are found on the presynaptic nerve terminals of neurons that secrete neurotransmitters such as GABA, dopamine, norepinephrine, and serotonin. A $GABA_b$ receptor agonist would inhibit the release of neurotransmitters. The benzodiazepine receptor, also called the omega receptor, is part of $GABA_a$. There is evidence that benzodiazepines increase the inhibitory effect of $GABA_a$ by increasing the affinity of $GABA_a$ receptors and thus prolonging the opening of the chloride channel.

Drug trials consistently show that benzodiazepines are better than placebo in treating anxiety disorders, but not all that much better. Reviews indicate that 55% of studies find an advantage for benzodiazepines over placebo. The real risk with benzodiazepine use is the rapidity with which drug dependence may occur. When benzodiazepines are used even for a brief period of time, a pattern of dependence and withdrawal often develops. The signs pointing to dependence and withdrawal are generally missed by the physician because they become part of the behavior and symptom complex for which the drug was originally prescribed. Shortness of breath, tachycardia, chest tightness, sweating, and stomach discomfort are frequently occurring anxiety symptoms that lead to a prescription of one of the benzodiazepines. These same symptoms, however, also characterize the withdrawal syndrome that accompanies benzodiazepine use. Other more general withdrawal symptoms that can occur include restlessness, agitation, irritability, and insomnia. Tyrer, Murphy, and Riley (1990) developed a questionnaire to assess the specific symptoms of benzodiazepine withdrawal. The most frequently reported symptoms, in rank order, were depression, noise sensitivity, shaking, muscle pains, dizziness, peculiar taste, pins and needles, light sensitivity, sore eyes, and feeling sick.

The shorter acting the drug, the quicker the onset of withdrawal symptoms. Anxiety patients given alprazolam (Xanax) for a period of a few weeks often cannot be withdrawn from the medication because of dependence Those who discontinue the drug may suffer rebound panic attacks worse than the panic attacks for which they had originally sought treatment. The percentage of patients who relapse following discontinuation of both short and long half-life benzodiazepines is very high.

Once a patient is drug-dependent, it is not possible to separate the symptoms for which the medication was prescribed from the symptoms associated with withdrawal. Physicians often base their judgment of the duration of estimated withdrawal solely in terms of the half-life of the medication. Thus, once the medication has cleared the body, they reason, there should be few if any symptoms due to withdrawal. For example, a patient with panic disorder controlled with Ativan or Xanax might be told to expect close to maximum chest pain, dizziness, and stomach distress immediately following termination of the benzodiazepine. These symptoms would be expected to quickly peak and, based solely on the understanding of the half-life of these drugs, disappear within 1 to 4 weeks. This is not the case: the symptoms often persist for months following drug discontinuation.

The persistence of withdrawal symptoms long after drug discontinuation indicates that variables other than the drug's half-life are controlling the symptoms. What happens in these circumstances is that the symptoms are usually viewed by both the patient and by the physician as a return of the anxiety condition rather than as signs of drug withdrawal, and so the medication cycle starts anew. Unfortunately, the patient is now using the medication to quiet withdrawal symptoms more than the original anxiety symptoms.

Attributing withdrawal symptoms solely to biochemical properties associated with the half-life of a drug fails to recognize the complex situational, psychological, and psychobiological determinants of drug withdrawal and what a patient needs to learn to get past these symptoms. Situational/environmental variables are extremely powerful determinants of drug withdrawal symptoms and are responsible for many incidences of relapse. The following clinical vignette describes an addict who is returning home after being withdrawn in a detoxification program from cocaine addiction:

> Harry turns onto the bridge that will take him back over to the old neighborhood. It feels good to be free again, and he hasn't used any heroin since he left the street for a 14-month stint in jail. No debts, no habit (the jail detox was harsh but is now long past), no problems. But as his wheels hit the rough surface of the bridge, his bowels begin to growl. As the skyline comes closer, he begins to yawn and his eyes water. He breaks out in sweat, gripping the wheel and trying to ignore the raw, acid taste in the back of his throat. He feels mounting panic, immediately recognizing this mouth-watery, nauseated feeling as the old sickness he left behind more than a year before. But here it is again. It *can't* be, but somehow it is. Muttering under his breath, Harry turns toward a familiar alley. He knows how to get rid of this sickness and fast. (Childress, Ehrman, Rohsenow, Robbins, & O'Brien, 1992, p. 56)

The situation facing the medical patient dependent on benzodiazepines is not significantly different from the plight facing Harry and other street-drug-dependent individuals. Anxiety, fear, and nervousness are symptom conditions that occur regularly in the context of daily living. Consequently, benzodiazepine medications that are used to alter or alleviate these psychobiological symptoms will become part of the stimulus complex that controls the very presence of these symptoms. Patients usually begin using an anxiolytic medication in order to sleep better, to socialize, or simply to get through specific times of the day. The regular use of medication in this fashion can very quickly become conditioned to cues in the natural environment and can activate very powerful withdrawal symptoms that are then mistakenly interpreted as a worsening of the condition for which the medication was prescribed:

> "The other night I went out to pick strawberries with a friend. Prior to going I decided not to take my anxiety medication, to see if I could manage without. I reasoned that I was with my friends, that nothing 'bad' was going to happen. After picking berries for a few minutes, I suddenly felt 'it' come over me—a lightheadedness and feeling that something was wrong. I said to myself, 'Oh no, not this time, you are not going to get me now.' I talked to myself, I talked

to my friend, and the symptom got worse. Finally I excused myself and took my medication—I immediately felt a bit better but the feeling did not last."

This individual's efforts to manage anxiety without medication are not that uncommon. She tried to fight the feelings for as long as she could but it is as if there is an inner realization that the struggle is doomed to fail and that medication will eventually be used. She had no realization of how to use her developing bodily sensations to lessen her dependency on medication. Instead, for her, the bodily sensations signified a desperate need for medication.

In clinical practice it is not always easy to anticipate the range of reactions that may occur during benzodiazepine withdrawal. Patients need to be prepared for a long and difficult struggle. Dependency reactions extend well beyond the period that the drugs have cleared the nervous system. Observe the experiences of a female patient who had been withdrawn from Xanax while in hospital for undiagnosed chest pain. She remained in hospital for a period sufficient for the Xanax to have cleared her body. Although she left the hospital feeling in good spirits, she became vulnerable to full-blown withdrawal symptoms at home:

"Some days are better than others. . . . At first, I thought I would be okay. . . . I felt better and I was trying to organize my life . . . I was doing fine and then one day I was in the kitchen, preparing dinner and 'bang' it just hit me . . . My chest started throbbing and I began wondering if it might be angina. I decided to ignore the tightness and keep working. I pushed my ribs together to ease the pain. . . . This seemed to help until I let go and then it returns. . . . At least I knew that it wasn't my heart . . . I went through the hospital program to get off medication, but I did not know that I would feel so bad. . . . It seemed as if my whole body was falling apart. . . . My physician was not available. . . . I started shaking. . . . I was a basket case, crying and no one was there to help so I decided I had to use Xanax. . . . I also decided at that point to never again considering stopping the Xanax. . . . I feel I can control the amount I use by slicing the pills in pieces. . . . I take a larger slice if I feel that I am going to fall apart."

There is no easy path to successful benzodiazepine withdrawal. Some physicians advocate slowly tapering the patient over a period of 6–8 weeks from the medication. This is often done by having patients alternate the days in which they take the drug (i.e., 1 day on medication and 1 day off medication). Another strategy involves substituting a longer acting benzodiazepine such as diazepam for a shorter acting agent such as alprazolam; the idea is to reduce the experience of "highs" and "lows" associated with the short-acting drug. Other drugs are often substituted, for example, an antidepressant or a "nonaddictive" anxiolytic such as buspar. But there is no evidence that drug substitution is effective. This strategy fails to recognize that drug dependency, once established, extends beyond the problematic drug in use. Recall from the list of commonalities of addiction the statement that *drug dependence is not inherently related to a given drug.* Substitution of another drug for benzodiazepine may lead to a relapse in the use of the first drug and/or dependence on the second drug. It is the *person* who becomes drug dependent and his/her dependency is often associated with a number of drugs. We might use an analogy to alcoholism: drug substitution strategies are similar to controlling drinking by slowly reducing the number of drinks consumed per day by substituting wine for a favorite scotch.

Benzodiazepine withdrawal is accompanied by amplification of the original somatic and cognitive anxiety symptoms as well as by the appearance of new symptoms, all of which make it extremely difficult for the individual to stop using the medication. The symptoms generally wax and wane and will vary in severity and type. Panic-based symptoms involving fear of choking, inability to sleep, nightmares, dysphoria, severe mood swings, irritability, and just plain "yuckiness" are commonly experienced, even when the benzodiazepines are withdrawn following a slow taper. The anticipation and fear of experiencing these symptoms makes it very hard for the patient to believe that he/she can manage without medication. Some form of adjuvant medication (e.g., an antidepressant, a major tranquilizer) may be temporarily required, but patients must be told that there are no drugs that can bypass the withdrawal syndrome.

The elderly patient who is benzodiazepine-dependent is especially difficult to treat. One hypothesis holds that both aging and unresolved stress resemble chronic benzodiazepine use in terms of several behavioral, biochemical, and neuroendocrinal phenomena. According to Lechin, van der Dijs, and Benaim (1996), normal aging, chronic benzodiazepine use, and unresolved stress are each associated with behavioral confusion, fatigue, dizziness, syncope, panic, and insomnia, and also with neuroendocrine depletion of noradrenaline, dopamine, serotonin, and cortisol. In their view, the elderly patient who is facing considerable stress should not be administered benzodiazepines, simply because its use will increase the patient's risk for the above symptom conditions as well as facilitate the onset of other acute and chronic disease conditions.

A study by Swinson and colleagues (Swinson, Cox, Shulman, Kuch, & Woszczyna, 1992) established how powerful anxiolytic medication can become in influencing the day-to-day behaviors of anxiety disorder patients. As part of a larger study, panic disorder patients with agoraphobia were asked to complete the Mobility Inventory (Chambless, Caputo, Jasin, Gracely, & Williams, 1985). The questionnaire identifies 28 situations that are potentially frightening to agoraphobic individuals. It includes enclosed places like theaters, supermarkets, tunnels, and restaurants; open spaces; riding in buses, subways, and planes; and situations such as being far away from home, standing in lines, and walking on the street. The usual format is to ask subjects to rate their anxiety in these situations when accompanied and when alone. In the Swinson et al. study the patients were also asked to rate their anxiety in these situations *when without* medication. The anxiety ratings were higher for every situation under the without medication condition when compared to the alone condition. The situations associated with the greatest fear of being without medication were: in an airplane, being far away from home, in a subway, at an auditorium or theater, and at a party or social gathering. These findings demonstrate how frightening the prospect of living without medication can become to the anxiety patient.

There are treatment programs that follow the principles of relapse prevention and utilize techniques of cognitive biobehavioral therapy to assist patients in the management of benzodiazepine withdrawal. These programs provide participants with a realistic understanding of the dangers of multiple drug use, the situational and psychosocial determinants of withdrawal, and the varied manner in which withdrawal symptoms occur. Patients are provided with cognitive and biobehavioral skills for managing the withdrawal symptoms. Otto et al. (1992) developed a program that integrates somatic awareness and cognitive behavioral coping strategies with the systematic tapering of benzodiazepine use. With alprazolam, for example, the dosage is reduced 0.25 mg every second day down to 2.0 mg and then 0.125 mg every second day thereafter. Over a course of 10 weekly sessions, patients are also taught to recognize the symptoms of withdrawal and to utilize both somatic awareness (muscle relaxation and diaphragmatic breathing) and cognitive coping strategies to modify their symptoms. Preliminary data indicated that 60% of a small sample provided with cognitive biobehavioral training and tapering remained free of benzodiazepines for at least 4 months. Less than 30% of the patients who underwent tapering alone were still off benzodiazepines during the follow-up period. It must be noted that the use of a 10-week tapering protocol is unduly long and costly if the patient is in hospital. However, it provides the patient with reassurance against experiencing full-blown "cold turkey" symptoms. The real difficulty is the last step: giving up the final pill. It is generally at this point that patients finally understand that they need to take a very active role in managing their somatic symptoms if they are to remain medication-free. To this point, they may have relied on the medication remaining to get them through the day and night.

Patients who are dependent on benzodiazepines can be extremely difficult to maintain free of drugs for long periods of time. There is no simple answer to preventing relapse; each case has to be approached separately. Treatment programs based on relapse prevention can be strengthened substantially by incorporating somatic awareness as a key if not the central focus of intervention. Anxiety disorder patients are especially frightened by the bodily symptoms of withdrawal, and cognitive strategies alone are often ineffective in dealing with such symptoms. Many patients are surprised about just how powerful chest tightness, dizziness, dyspnea, and other physical symptoms can become during periods of withdrawal. They are also surprised to discover just how long it can take before these symptoms begin to lessen in intensity.

Individuals who are dependent on anxiolytics have learned to rely on medication to deal with the anxieties and pressures of work, family, friends, and life itself. Marital and family issues are often paramount and there is often an impatience from family members regarding the patient's "lack of will" and "unwillingness to change." Quite often the drug-dependent individual feels that there is no spousal support for change. If anything, such a perceived lack of caring provides a good reason for the continued use of medication. Sometimes it is appropriate to include a family member in the treatment plan and sometimes it is not appropriate. In either case, stressful family encounters are utilized in therapy as a risk factor during which the patient needs to be especially aware of the appearance and/or worsening of somatic symptoms. Once identified, these symptoms are worked through in the context of ongoing somatic awareness training. If a patient comes to recognize that he/she is at risk for symptom exacerbation in the presence of a particular family circumstance, he/she can begin to take steps to prevent the onset or worsening of the symptom by avoiding the circumstance or by self-regulating bodily reactions when faced with the situation.

It is important to encourage patients to praise themselves for altering thoughts and feelings associated with symptoms. Self-praise is a very important aspect of helping patients deal with withdrawal. These individuals feel that they are close to becoming out of control, and they can experience fear of "going mad" over their symptoms. It is a very fine line between feelings of "losing it" and maintaining symptom control during periods of intense withdrawal. Patients often ignore or overlook successes and so need to be repeatedly reminded that the management of psychobiological processes associated with drug dependency represents the most difficult personal task they have ever undertaken. They need to engage in self-praise on a day-to-day, if not on an hour-to-hour, basis as they slowly experience the bodily changes associated with mastery of the withdrawal syndrome. Therapists need to be supportive during setbacks and encouraging during successes.

CHRONIC PAIN AND THE CODEINE DANCE

Codeine is generally considered a safe and effective prescription analgesic for controlling chronic pain disorders. Codeine-based analgesics are not viewed with the same addictive concern as the stronger narcotic medications such as morphine. However, this view is changing as the drug-dependency risks of prolonged codeine use are becoming better recognized. Even more problematic is the suspicion that the overuse of codeine medication can actually worsen chronic benign pain conditions. We now know in regard to benzodiazepines that long-term use of these drugs may establish a withdrawal condition characterized by anxiety symptoms that are worse than the original anxiety symptoms for which the drug was prescribed. The same is true for codeine and other analgesics that are used for the control of chronic pain. Long-term use of codeine can lead to a worsening of the underlying chronic pain condition. The dance metaphor in the title of this section was deliberately chosen to capture the complex psychobiological, situational, and interpersonal issues involved in habilitating the codeine-dependent pain patient.

Codeine, a member of the opioid analgesic class of drugs, is the pain-relieving agent found in a number of analgesic medications. The opioid analgesics are a group of drugs that resemble morphine in their actions on the body. Morphine and codeine are the two natural pain-relieving agents found in opium. Morphine is by far the more potent of the two. An equivalent dose of codeine has one-tenth the analgesic efficacy of a dose of morphine. No other compounds are as effective as morphine and codeine in the control of pain. But no other compounds cause as much difficulty in terms of patient abuse. Although codeine is viewed as a much less addictively dangerous compound than morphine, its regular use can result in a number of complicated and difficult-to-manage medical and behavioral health problems. Codeine can become a way of life for many individuals with a use for managing distress that extends well beyond physical pain.

The choice of opioid for the control of chronic nonmalignant pain is based on the *analgesic ladder* concept adopted by the World Health Organization Expert Committee (1990). The first rung on the ladder represents the use of nonopioids such as acetaminophen alone or acetaminophen in combination with a nonsteroidal anti-inflammatory drug. The second rung of the ladder involves the administration of one of the weaker opioids, consisting of a product containing acetaminophen or aspirin plus either codeine (Fiorinal C) or oxycodone (Percocet). Codeine is the most commonly used opioid in medicine. There is now a controlled-release codeine preparation that lasts 12 hours and is advertised as providing "around-the-clock pain control." If codeine fails to control the pain, the patient is moved to the third rung of the ladder by being switched to one of the "strong opioids," usually oxycodone, morphine, or hydromorphone. One milligram of oxycodone is considered equivalent to 10 mg of codeine. Hydromorphone (Dilaudid) has an especially high affinity for opioid receptors and is reported to be 7 to 12 times more potent than morphine. Morphine is currently the preferred opioid, especially because it can also be given in long-acting form (MS Contin).

Opioid receptors are found throughout the brain and spinal cord, in the neural plexus of the gastrointestinal tract, in parts of the autonomic nervous system, and on white cells (Jaffe, 1992). Opioid receptors are found in highest concentrations in the limbic regions of the brain (Julien, 1995). There are a number of different types of opioid receptors; the major types are called *mu, kappa,* and *delta* receptors. Activation of the mu receptors is believed to be responsible for the analgesic properties and the dependency problems of morphine and codeine. Codeine is initially inactive as an opioid and is able to activate mu receptors only after it is metabolized by the body and converted to morphine. If this conversion does not occur, codeine very quickly loses its analgesic effect for that individual.

Energizing Properties

Codeine, like morphine, is often taken for its ability to produce positive feelings of energy and well-being. It may come as a surprise that the regular use of codeine for pain can acquire significant influence over a person's emotional behavior and sense of control. Codeine can be used not only for its analgesic effect on bodily pain but for its ability to *energize* and alleviate feelings of depression and boredom. This additional quality of codeine is seldom mentioned but represents a significant component of continued codeine use. Patients who rely on codeine for its uplifting properties will seldom acknowledge to their physician that they are using the drug in this fashion. However, there are many instances where the positive mood attributes of codeine use outweigh its analgesic benefits for the patient.

The energizing and other positive reinforcement capabilities of opioids are mediated through the brain's dopamine reward system. The ventral tegmentum and associated substantia nigra are midbrain nuclei that are part of the brain dopamine reward system. The nucleus acumbens is considered to be the center of the dopamine circuit. GABA inhibitory interneurons in the dopamine system are attached to mu-opioid receptors (Julien, 1995). Activation of the mu-receptors increases the outward flow of potassium ions (K+), leading to hyperpolarization of the GABA interneurons. The GABA interneurons, being hyperpolarized, have a reduced inhibitory effect on the dopamine neurons, resulting in increased excitability of the dopamine system.

Opioids also have anxiolytic properties. Codeine and morphine have emotional quieting properties, which results in their use for the management of emotional pain as well as physical pain. In some instances the effect can be associated with a form of "mental clouding" characterized by lack of concentration, apathy, lethargy, and a sense of tranquillity. For some individuals, codeine and other opioids have the capacity to alleviate depression, reduce anxiety, and inhibit feelings of general distress (Jaffe, 1992). The inhibitory action of opioids on GABA neurons likely accounts for their anxiolytic action. In this case, the primary site of action is the locus coeruleus, the main clustering of norepinephrine neurons in the brain. Many patients who are dependent on codeine are also dependent on benzodiazepines, especially the short-acting benzodiazepines. Given that opioids, with a biological half-life of 2 hours, are metabolized very rapidly, there is the potential for a very powerful withdrawal response in the patient who is using both short-acting benzodiazepines and opioids on approximately the same administration schedule.

The fact that the benefits of codeine extend beyond analgesia to include the activation of positive feelings and the quieting of negative feelings makes codeine dependency a complex and powerful force to contend with in therapy. Codeine use, at least for some individuals, provides the means of control over all forms of emotional suffering. For such patients, any attempt to withdraw medication without the patient's full participation is not likely to be successful.

Withdrawal and drug-seeking behaviors associated with codeine dependency generally go unnoticed and untreated on hospital wards. These patients have generally been admitted for the management of some chronic medical condition, and analgesics with codeine are generally given without much attention or concern. If codeine dependency is suspected, the patient may be switched to a nonopioid analgesic without concern or development of a treatment plan to deal with possible withdrawal symptoms. A standard intervention in cases of suspected codeine dependency is to switch the patient from the opioid containing codeine (e.g., Tylenol #3) to an analgesic without codeine such as acetaminophen (Tylenol ES). From a pharmacological perspective, the shift from opioid to nonopioid medication is seen as straightforward. Given that opioids have a short biological half-life of 2–3 hours, it is reasoned that the receptors should be drug-free relatively quickly and peak withdrawal symptoms should begin to subside within 5–7 days.

The expectation of relatively brief and innocuous withdrawal symptoms works best for minor physiological responses following short-term opioid use, such as temperature change, sweating, and pupillary size (Jaffe, 1992). Withdrawal is far more complex in individuals who have engaged in long-term opioid use. The symptoms and symptom determinants are psychobiological as well as physiological in nature and include frightening throat spasms, uncontrollable coughing, nausea, panic anxiety, depression, insomnia, and severe abdominal aches and pains. These withdrawal symptoms may persist for weeks, months, or in some cases years. Explanations based solely on the biological half-life of drug molecules cannot explain the dramatic and persistent nature of codeine-based withdrawal symptoms.

In order to understand the experiential aspects of codeine withdrawal, consider the description provided by a 62-year-old patient who was admitted to a psychiatry unit for multiple drug dependencies, including codeine, benzodiazepine, and ergotamine (ergotamine is a vasodilator used in the prophylaxis of migraine). During a 1-week hospitalization period, the patient was withdrawn from all codeine and benzodiazepine. The codeine was replaced with acetaminophen (Tylenol ES), and the SSRI antidepressant Paxil was also prescribed by the attending psychiatrist. The following represents her description of the subjective changes she experienced following discharge:

"It was too easy. . . . It was very strange . . . I stopped all this medication and I was out in a week. There was something wrong. Whether I coasted with the amounts of codeine I had in me . . . then boom . . . the anxiety went wild. My head hurt, my throat was

tight, I was scared. . . . My mind said, 'Take a pill, take a pill . . . this
is silly to suffer.' I was full of Tylenol ES. . . . I still find it ridiculous
that I am taking this Mickey Mouse pill when I used to take hand-
fuls of codeine. I got to think of it as codeine. I still have places in
the cupboards where my Tylenol is sitting in the same place as I
used to keep my codeine. There are days when I say to myself,
'This is so painful—wouldn't it make sense to take codeine until
you die. It's probably going to kill you anyway.' I am really fed up—
last night I thought I would get away from it all by going to sleep. I
woke up from dreaming of pills, of all kinds, pills I don't think of
when I am awake."

Central Nervous System Plasticity

Biochemical pain researchers now suspect that the long-term use
of codeine contributes to functional changes within the central nervous
system (CNS). These changes are discussed under the general concept
of CNS *plasticity*. The concept of CNS plasticity was developed to
explain the persistence of pathological pain after the healing of dam-
aged tissue. It is believed that the persistent pain results both from a
reduction in the threshold of peripheral nociceptors and from an
increase in the excitability of CNS neurons involved in pain transmis-
sion. The net effect of these changes is to lead to a condition of
hyperalgesia as well as allodynia and persistent pain. "Hyperalgesia" is
defined by the International Association for the Study of Pain (http://
weber.u.washington.edu/~crc/IASP.html) as an increased response to
a stimulus that is normally painful; "allodynia" is defined as pain due
to a stimulus that does not normally provoke pain. Allodynia involves a
change in the quality of sensation in that the original response to the
stimulus may have been touch, warmth, or some other sensation rather
than pain.

The suggestion being made is that the sensory changes that accompany long-term use of opioid analgesics are mediated by biochemical
events that extend well beyond the interaction of the opioid molecule
with the opioid receptor. Chronic exposure to opioids can result in significant biochemical and molecular changes within the CNS itself. At the
center of these CNS changes is the N-methyl-D-aspartate (NMDA) receptor (Mao, Price, & Mayer, 1995). NMDA is an excitatory amino acid
receptor. Changes in the NMDA receptor following prolonged opioid
use are believed to contribute to both opioid tolerance and withdrawal.
Investigators suspect that the NMDA excitatory receptor plays a role in
the phenomenon of *physiological wind up*. Wind up is a form of increased

CNS sensitivity whereby injury to a peripheral nerve leads to a progressive increase of response of dorsal horn cells in the spinal cord as well as a persistence of response in these cells for long periods after the stimulation ceases (McMahon, Lewin, & Wall, 1993). Other changes include an expansion of the dorsal horn receptive field and a lowering of stimulus threshold. All these changes taken together are used to account for pain states associated with hyperalgesia and allodynia. The biochemical processes involved are complex and involve enhanced synaptic efficacy combined with reduced efficacy of the opioid receptor-channel complex and/or opioid receptor-associated second-messenger systems (Mao et al., 1995).

The NMDA receptor research examining opioid tolerance and withdrawal is preliminary, but serves to reinforce clinical suspicions that all is not well with the strategy of long-term use of opioids for controlling chronic benign pain. In addition to the problem of tolerance, many pain patients using opioids continue to suffer from pain as well as to show evidence of drug dependency and drug withdrawal. This is a difficult problem, especially when the pain experienced combines with the distress of opioid withdrawal to produce an even more severe and complicated state of central sensitivity and psychological suffering.

> The lack of efficacy of opioids after chronic use may not only be due to changes secondary to the use of the opioid, but also to the fact that these changes are *exacerbated by the inputs associated with the pain itself.* The clinicians then are faced with a difficult Hobson's Choice [a situation in which an apparently free choice is given when there is no real alternative]. On the one hand, they wish to intervene and reduce the pain; on the other hand, the continued intervention may reduce the likelihood of long-term control. If persistent pain (i.e., injury) contributes to the lack of efficacy of the opioid, the problem is made even worse. (Basbaum, 1995, p. 349; emphasis added)

We cannot say at this time if physiological wind-up is part of the puzzle in explaining codeine dependence, but the fact that physiochemical processes beyond the receptor–drug molecule interaction are being implicated indicates that the CNS is heavily involved. With the involvement of the CNS comes the patient's understanding and experiencing of the varied physiological symptoms that occur during codeine withdrawal. Very frightening physical symptoms occur, and these symptoms cannot be readily ignored. Throat tightness, for example, may signify to the patient that he/she will soon be unable to breathe. A similar psychobiological link may exist between codeine withdrawal and chronic daily headache.

Analgesic-Induced Pain Disorders

The observation that many forms of chronic pain remain uncontrolled with continued analgesic use has generally been attributed to a worsening or progression of underlying disease conditions rather than to analgesic use per se. It is only recently that the determinants of chronic benign pain syndromes have been extended to include analgesics themselves. Headache experts are familiar with the analgesic-withdrawal headache, a variant of chronic daily headache that occurs in association with prolonged analgesic use, especially codeine use. Chronic headache generally occurs on a daily or near-daily basis. Individuals who suffer chronic headaches are particularly prone to using large quantities of analgesic medications. The most frequently used prescription analgesic by these individuals is acetaminophen with codeine; its use is known to increase with both age and number of experienced headache days (Von Korff, Galer, & Stang, 1995). The issue is usually raised whether the medication is causing the headache or the headache is causing the use of medication. It is known that cessation of headache medications leads to symptoms similar to those associated with codeine withdrawal (i.e., headache, nausea, cramps, diarrhea, sleeplessness, emotional distress).

Chronic daily headache is extremely difficult to manage. Biobehavioral interventions involving relaxation training, biofeedback, and cognitive therapy, although routinely utilized in headache clinics, are not effective with this group. Several studies have found that chronic daily headache sufferers are poor candidates for biobehavioral treatments, showing improvement rates of less than 15% (Bakal, Demjen, & Duckro, 1994). There is a strong likelihood that poor responders are more likely to be dependent on analgesic medication. Thus, interventions that focus directly on eliminating the use of analgesics may be more effective than interventions that deal with the biobehavioral management of headache symptoms.

There is some research showing that the withdrawal of analgesic medications is associated with reduction of headache activity (Cantwell-Simmons, Duckro, & Richardson, 1993). However, these studies have generally replaced the analgesic medication with another medication or have not provided the headache sufferers with alternatives for managing their condition. Diener et al. (1989) followed 139 patients with chronic daily headache who were withdrawn from medications in hospital over a 2-week period. At discharge, 45% of the patients were headache-free. However, at a mean 2.9-year follow-up, the improvement rate dropped considerably. Moreover, the majority of these patients continued to use some form of medication, although at reduced levels. It is possible that the fear of experiencing even worse pain without medication resulted in the resumption of medication use. These patients were not provided with alternate strategies for managing their headache in their home environment.

Other pain symptoms beyond the original problem may develop in association with long-term codeine use. An especially problematic and frightening withdrawal symptom experienced by codeine users is abdominal pain. Patients often describe this pain as persistent in nature, although they will acknowledge that it is temporarily relieved with codeine and/or other opioids. Patients have difficulty describing the exact nature and location of the pain beyond signifying the abdominal region. They also exhibit considerable psychological distress, insisting that they need something to control the pain. Their description is very suggestion of a pain condition with a large emotional/physiological withdrawal component. The pain, although unremitting, definitely increases in intensity as the usual time of medication dosing approaches.

These patients represent a management nightmare, especially for emergency room physicians. No matter how many previous investigations have been performed, there is always the remote possibility that an undetected organic disease is responsible for the patient's pain. Thus, they are required to investigate symptom complaints such as abdominal pain for medical causes, no matter how often the patient presents with the same symptom. Patients with chronic abdominal pain complaints have generally received numerous physical investigations involving ultrasound, endoscopy, and gastroscopy as a consequence of their repeated presentations to hospital or clinic. Elderly patients are especially difficult to diagnose because they present with a number of chronic disease conditions that may be exacerbating the abdominal pain. Unstable angina, duodenal or peptic ulcer, osteoporosis, osteoarthritis, rheumatoid arthritis, herpes zoster, and diverticulitis, represent some of the conditions that may be perceived as causing the pain. These are chronic disease conditions that are treated symptomatically, which means that patients are given a few days hospital rest while investigations are completed; medicated with sufficient opioids and benzodiazepines to control their pain, anxiety, and insomnia; and discharged to the care of their family physician.

A diagnosis of codeine–opioid dependency is difficult to make and can only be made on an exclusionary basis, that is, after all medical factors are ruled out. For this reason, the diagnosis of *abdominal pain not-yet-diagnosed* is often chosen to safeguard against the possibility that an organic cause of the pain has escaped detection. However, no matter how many investigations prove negative, codeine is seldom implicated as causing the symptoms and the patient is usually sent home with his/her codeine prescription intact—along with additional medication for stomach distress. A diagnosis indicative of chronic gastrointestinal sensitivity, such as lactose intolerance, irritable bowel, or spastic colon, may be made. Symptomatic relief, if it occurs, is usually short-lived; both the pain and the patient eventually return for treatment; and the investigative exercise is repeated. Codeine dependency should be considered as the primary problem in patients who use excessive codeine and who repeatedly present to clinics and/or hospital emergency departments with unexplained abdominal pain.

It is surprising that opioids are not suspected more frequently as the culprit in cases of unexplained stomach pain. Opium, which has constipating power, has been used throughout history to combat diarrhea. Indeed, opioid drugs are still key therapeutic agents in the treatment of diarrhea. Loperamide (Imodium) is a specialized opioid that can be sold without prescription because its action is primarily on the gut without getting into the CNS (Jaffe, 1992). Opioids cause intestinal tone to increase and motility to decrease, feces to dehydrate, and intestinal spasm to occur. The combination of these effects is what produces constipation. Drug withdrawal is associated with the opposite gastrointestinal activity and may explain the nonspecific cramps and pain these individuals report. A long history of codeine use (as well as use of other drugs) is generally noted on the medical chart of these difficult patients but the possibility that codeine withdrawal is responsible for the pain is not considered.

Sometimes physicians do recognize that opioids are part of the problem and that opioid discontinuation is part of the solution. However, their recommendations to the patient to reduce the use of codeine-based analgesics are politely ignored. Patients will insist that they need the codeine medication at home to control their pain. Even though they recognize that the codeine is not providing pain relief, they feel that their pain would be much worse without it. They have difficulty with the notion that the codeine is actually responsible for their ongoing pain and suffering.

The drug-seeking behaviors of a codeine-dependent pain patient are illustrated in the following medical chart segment. The patient was being weaned from codeine medication. During this particular charting period she was receiving a spasmolytic (Buscopan) as a substitute for codeine medication.

0620: Pt reports sleeping poorly, given Buscopan 10 mg for abdominal discomfort.

0915: Pt given whirlpool bath to aid in alleviating arthritic discomfort—bath effective in alleviating pain.

1000: Pt given Buscopan 10 mg for abdominal discomfort.

1100: Serax 15 mg given for agitation.

1300: Pt given Buscopan for pain.

1330: Pt required much encouragement to go outdoors. She finally agreed, but when she returned she was dizzy and weak—asked for Buscopan.

1440: Pt expressing concern about what quality of life will be like without codeine.

1630: Buscopan 10 mg given PRN.

1830: Pt called staff from washroom—took a nitro tablet for chest tightness—sitting on toilet holding nitro spray "just in case."

The same pattern of drug-seeking behavior and pain complaints continued throughout the entire period of the patient's admission, in spite of the fact that several different substitute medications for codeine were attempted for pain control. The patient had used opioid medication for at least 30 years and was frightened at the prospect of losing control and becoming depressed if she tried to manage without medication. She resumed codeine following discharge, stating that it was too late for her to change.

In this case, the patient did not participate in the decision to remove the opioid from her drug regimen as the attending physician simply decided that opioid discontinuation would be in her best interest. Patients *must* be made part of the decision-making process when they are about to be withdrawn from an addictive medication. They have to be ready to change, and they have to be provided with strategies and skills for dealing with the withdrawal symptoms that are going to occur. In many cases, they are simply overwhelmed by the withdrawal symptoms and experiences and consequently resume use of their medication.

Inpatient pain programs generally recommend that opioids should be administered on an "around the clock" dosing to avoid creating a contingency between pain behaviors and opioid administration. The patient in the case described above was receiving Buscopan on a PRN, or "as-needed," schedule. The standard prescription PRN order can lead patients to verbalize excessive distress and suffering in order to get their medication. Even when medication is administered "by the clock," physicians will usually add an "as needed" dosing to deal with so-called breakthrough pain. Neither of these drug administration schedules solves the problem of dependency. Making the medication time-contingent rather than pain-complaint-contingent does not solve the problem because patients will continue to exhibit increased distress and pain as the time of dosing approaches. Worse yet, the very behaviors that the medication is designed to control, such as abdominal pain, may now result from the developing withdrawal syndrome as the plasma drug concentration diminishes following the last administrations. It is not uncommon to find patients who report that their pain increases in intensity as the time of the next scheduled dosing approaches. Patients will line up at the nursing station in anticipation of the next drug administration.

The common practice of treating codeine or opioid withdrawal by substituting an nonopioid analgesic for the opioid analgesic, although sometimes effective, is not without risk. In the above case study, the patient was given a spasmolytic as a substitute for codeine, presumably to ease the discomfort of abdominal pain during withdrawal from codeine. However, this patient was highly drug-dependent; the dependency extended beyond codeine to include all medications that she might use for pain and abdominal distress. The phrase "a rose is a rose is a rose" comes to mind to capture the difficulties associated with attempting to treat drug dependency through drug substitution. With this patient, her withdrawal symptoms are no longer simply under the control of codeine. The substitute medication was alleviating the abdominal distress but was also maintaining the drug dependency. Her repeated pleas for "something" to relieve the pain and distress emphasize that for many chronic conditions drug dependency is not inherently related to a given drug.

Nonopioid substitute medications for pain control are generally less effective than opioids in alleviating withdrawal symptoms. Patients who are switched to acetaminophen for pain control after a long history of codeine use often complain that the acetaminophen "is like popping candy." Still, they continue to use the substitute, rationalizing that it is better than nothing. Substitute medication provides short-term symptom relief but removes the patient from having to deal with the dependency issue. Effective treatment can require the removal of all medications that might be sustaining the withdrawal symptom complex.

A patient who had discontinued codeine use complained of withdrawal symptoms involving throat tightness, insomnia, shortness of breath, and panic anxiety for several months following discontinuation of codeine. It was discovered that she was using 8–12 acetaminophen a day as a substitute for codeine. She was asked to discontinue the acetaminophen, but the withdrawal symptoms continued. It was discovered that she continued to carry two acetaminophen tablets in her purse just in case she felt that she was "going to go crazy." Although not using analgesic medication, she had created a cycle of perverse logic that in fact was maintaining her medication dependence. The withdrawal symptoms only began to decrease when she stopped carrying or handling medication and mastered her fear of being entirely without pills.

Fear of Suffering and Depression

Codeine dependency also has a very significant cognitive component. Codeine is often used to control mood as well as pain, and therefore it is not surprising that codeine-dependent patients are intensely afraid of the prospect of having to live without the drug. Codeine dependency can be conceptualized at the cognitive level as a form of *fear of suffering*. The fear of fear concept was originally proposed for understanding the symptoms of panic disorder and agoraphobia (Goldstein & Chambless, 1978). Panic symptoms are maintained largely because the individual develops a fear of the bodily sensations associated with panic attacks. Biological vulnerability toward anxious apprehension sets the stage for the disorder, but once it develops the individual becomes afraid of the anxiety itself, hence the fear of fear. The beginning episodes of the disorder might be marked by a predominance of somatic symptoms such as heart palpitations, chest pressure, shortness of breath, dizziness, dry throat, and nausea. As the disorder becomes more entrenched, the individual becomes afraid of the symptoms themselves and the situations in which they occur. Common fears they experience include going crazy, having a heart attack, or losing control.

Codeine-dependent patients exhibit a very similar fear, but it extends beyond the experience of pain to include suffering as well as depression. Their thinking is dominated by fears of being without medication. Thoughts such as "I need something," "Why should I suffer," and "I can't stand this" are very prevalent prior to ingesting codeine. Many patients are unwilling to consider life without codeine; they fear that without the medication their situation will be intolerable. For others, the dependency on medication is "proof" that they have "real pain" and need ongoing medical treatment. Many also have a deep fear of not being able to sleep without the analgesic. For many patients, the fear of suffering exceeds the fear of pain itself.

The distinction between *pain* and *suffering* is clinically important for understanding the codeine-dependent patient. The International

Association for the Study of Pain (Merskey & Bogduk, 1994) defines "pain" as "an unpleasant sensory and emotional experience associated with actual or potential tissue damage, or described in terms of such damage." "Suffering" is defined as a state of emotional distress that may or may not coexist with actual pain. Suffering has been characterized as occurring "when we assess ourselves in a situation and don't like where we are, where we have been, or where we are going *and* we can take no actions to close this gap" (Fordyce, 1995, p. 14). This description, which resembles characterizations of depression and hopelessness, is intended to capture the affective responses to bodily pain.

Suffering in the form of dissatisfaction or unhappiness may have been lurking in the background at the time the pain problem and codeine use began. Now with the prospect of increased pain and distress as a consequence of codeine withdrawal, the patient may anticipate suffering that will be too much to bear. Many patients fear coming off codeine not so much because of anticipated pain but because of a an apprehension that their "world will come apart." Pain is no longer the central issue in their fear. The notion that pain and suffering are related but distinct dimensions of the chronic pain experience reflects the fact that pain itself, as noted in the definition, is more than a primary sensation. Pain cannot be viewed as a sensation in the same way that taste, vision, smell, and touch are viewed as sensations.

The observation that suffering and depression coexist in pain patients makes it difficult to decide whether the depression should be treated as a separate clinical condition. Some psychiatrists interpret codeine dependence as secondary to psychiatric issues surrounding depression and recommend that the depression should be treated with medication during the period of codeine withdrawal. A common practice is to prescribe one of the SSRI antidepressants, such as paroxetine (Paxil), during the codeine withdrawal period. The assumption is that the SSRIs have low pharmacological dependence potential and do not add to the risk of codeine dependence. There is a danger, however, in adding to the withdrawal syndrome at the behavioral level because the patient will continue to believe that some form of "quick fix" can be achieved by using medication to avoid the intensity of drug cravings and withdrawal symptoms. Another possibility is that the depression is actually the *result of* rather than the *cause of* codeine use and withdrawal. That is, the patient may be experiencing a multitude of somatic symptoms during withdrawal that serve as triggers for episodes of negative mood and depression. The negative feelings may in large part reflect the patient's realization that there is no medication he/she can use to feel better. In these instances, providing the patient with some relief through the use of antidepressant medication would add to the dependency problem and increase the probability of patient relapse for codeine.

How does one determine whether depression should or should not be treated with medication in the codeine-dependent pain patient? Although this question has not been addressed directly, the larger issue of whether depression contributes to or results from chronic pain has been examined many times. Reviews of the literature have repeatedly observed an elevated rate of depression among chronic pain patients. An estimated 30–54% of chronic pain patients meet psychiatric diagnostic criteria for major depressive disorder (Banks & Kerns, 1996). There is uncertainty about whether the depression causes the pain, the depression results from the pain, or the pain and depression occur concomitantly. Overall, the available evidence seems to be more consistent with the hypothesis that depression results from living with years of pain. As a symptom, pain is somewhat unique in its ability to pervade consciousness and interfere with cognitive and emotional functioning. Unremitting pain can undermine the patient's hope for a better future. Although chronic pain may not inspire fears of dying, it can create a pervasive sense of hopelessness—a fear that the pain will never improve, a fear that the pain will worsen, and a fear of progressive impairment.

The following clinical case illustrates the complex processes that determine a patient's psychological state during withdrawal. Earlier I presented the case of a patient who was struggling with withdrawal following the substitution of acetaminophen for codeine. In the following clinical excerpt, she describes the emotional suffering and depression that occur in the absence of codeine:

"I have got too many feelings. This is just too much—I don't want to think about myself and my life. Maybe this is why I have been taking drugs all along. I don't want to think about all this. This week my marriage nearly ended. My husband has spent a whole life convincing me how unimportant I am. There was a hockey game on television. I was feeling bad and my husband said, 'If the game bothers you I will turn it off.' Normally, I would have said, 'Never mind, watch the game,' but this time I said, 'Why don't we watch another channel?' He replied, 'You mean I cannot watch the hockey game?' Here I am feeling like I might die and this man says 'Can't I watch the hockey game'! I suddenly realized how much anger and resentment I harbored within myself. When I was a young mother, with two children, I was left to fend for myself, and now that's all stirred back up. . . . "

Is this patient's depression causing the pain and withdrawal or is her pain and withdrawal causing the depression? There is probably not a definitive answer to this question, other than that depression is likely both a cause and an effect of the pain. Viewed from a systems perspective, the direction of causality becomes circular and bidirectional, with depression contributing to and resulting from ongoing pain and depression. It is best to accept the depression, resentment, anger, and pain as components of a larger suffering complex associated with drug withdrawal. Negative feelings toward her spouse, for example, may have become salient because of the withdrawal from codeine and other medications. These symptoms, although originating early in her relationship, are best conceptualized as a symptom occurring in the absence of codeine. The systems perspective would not automatically provide depression with causal status during withdrawal and would not suggest the use of additional medication. The administration of an antidepressant runs the risk of reinforcing drug dependency and making withdrawal from codeine more rather than less difficult.

There is a need for clinical observation and outcome research to determine whether the administration of an antidepressant during codeine withdrawal is harmful or helpful. Caution must always be used in giving a drug of any kind to a patient who is struggling to control the cravings for codeine. In theory, the ideal treatment situation is to have codeine-dependent patients discontinue all medication for pain and other symptoms that are not life-threatening. This step is seldom taken, but should be encouraged. The psychobiological and interpersonal changes that occur in individuals who discontinue all mood and analgesic medication can be remarkable:

A 70-year-old woman presented to the emergency room complaining of abdominal pain. The patient had a history of peptic ulcer and irritable bowel disease. She located the pain in the right quadrant of her stomach and noted that at times it felt as if it was radiating from her back. She also suffered from osteoporosis and arthritis of the legs and feet. She had a fear of falling, although there was no history of falls. The patient showed some evidence of depressed mood as well as an anticipatory worry that something bad was going to happen to her or to a family member. She had little energy, had difficulty getting out of bed each morning, and preferred to stay at home rather than do things in the community or visit with family. She had experienced a number of family losses due to heart disease and cancer. Her most recent loss was her husband, who had succumbed to heart failure after a lengthy illness. The patient relied heavily on codeine-based medications for abdominal and lower back pain control and for general *energy* to face the day. She also used a number of over-the-counter and prescription gastrointestinal medications.

During several emergency admissions the patient received thorough gastrointestinal medical work-ups that included a gastroscopy, an endoscopy, and an abdominal ultrasound. Each time the investigations revealed a normal esophogus, a normal duodenum, and no significant evidence of organicity. Over the various admissions a number of tentative diagnoses were made, including recurrent peptic ulcer disease, epigastric pain, abdominal pain not-yet-diagnosed, urinary tract infection, syncope, depression, diverticulosis, unstable angina, and early dementia. The dementia diagnosis was based on the observation by psychiatrists that the patient appeared confused and disoriented. She also had difficulty with the Mini-Mental Status exam. For example, she could not draw a clock with the hands at "10 minutes after 11," producing instead one hand at 10 and one hand at 11. She could not perform the serial 7's task and also perseverated with her speech by repeating rather than answering questions.

With each admission, the attending physician noted the patient's long-standing use of codeine but it was never stated that her subjective and physical symptoms might be the result of the codeine use. This possibility was finally considered and the patient was admitted to a geriatric inpatient "survival without inpatient medication" (SWIM) program and over 6 weeks gradually withdrawn from codeine medication. At first the codeine was substituted with a plain analgesic but her abdominal symptoms continued to persist. Finally the patient agreed with a decision to withdraw from all analgesic and stomach medications. She was encouraged to manage her pain and stomach distress with relaxation. After 6 weeks in hospital she was much improved but found the symptoms returned upon returning home. She had to learn to live without medication for the first time in 40 years. The patient had used codeine for this period not simply to control pain but to provide her with the energy to live. Two years after using her last analgesic, she still awakened each morning with mild abdominal distress and the cognition of needing some codeine to feel better. However, the abdominal symptoms and drug-seeking thoughts have disappeared, although getting out of bed each day remains a struggle. The patient has regained her cognitive faculties, remains anxious when she leaves her home but actively does participate in community and family activities. She has no abdominal symptoms or pain and although she has minor back pain in the morning she has no plan to use analgesics to obtain relief.

This patient, unlike other examples, was ready to participate in a full withdrawal program. Her readiness, however, was not immediate and had to be nurtured through a number of preliminary interventions designed to prepare her for withdrawal. Prochaska's (1995) stages of change model is useful to keep in mind when attempting codeine withdrawal programs. Prochaska's model depicts behavioral change in lifestyle as consisting of six stages: precontemplation, contemplation, preparation, action, maintenance, and termination. During the precontemplative stage, this patient believed that her abdominal pain was due to reactivation of peptic ulcer disease and/or lactose intolerance. Considerable therapeutic effort from members of a multidisciplinary team was required to have her begin contemplating codeine discontinuation and to finally take action to quit all analgesic medication. Furthermore, a form of maintenance or relapse prevention was added to her discontinuation through community participation in a senior's program.

The discussion of codeine dependency and codeine withdrawal is intended to caution rather than scare people about the use of opioids for the management of pain. In the acute situation, codeine represents an extremely useful analgesic for controlling pain. There are also individuals who use codeine to manage chronic pain and who do not exhibit psychobiological signs of dependency. There are others who are able to terminate opioid use of all kinds, remain on nonopioid analgesics, and live a normal life. Codeine use, however, can easily get out of control and create a myriad of difficult-to-manage symptoms and health problems. Codeine even in small doses can become associated with powerful physical and psychological behaviors that maintain rather than reduce pain and emotional suffering.

Opioids are receiving increased scrutiny in terms of their efficacy and effectiveness in controlling chronic pain. There is a general agreement that with cancer pain, long-term use of opioids remains the treatment of choice (Portenoy, 1996). Opioid treatment can provide relief to 70–90% of patients, and there is little concern being expressed about addiction or drug dependency among cancer patients. Indeed, the World Health Organization stresses that opioids should be used more frequently to manage cancer pain. The same organization says little with respect to opioids and benign chronic pain. In fact, the utility of opioids in managing noncancer chronic pain is being challenged in both basic and applied research. Basic research, as indicated earlier, is beginning to suggest that prolonged opioid use may lead to functional changes in the nervous system that contribute to drug tolerance, drug withdrawal, and increased pain sensitivity.

There are those who continue to insist that opioid dependence is a rare event in medical settings and only occurs in those individuals who have a history of psychological disturbance or drug dependence. Melzack (1990b), for example, believes that fears of widespread opioid addiction are unfounded. He referred to a study involving 11,882 hospital inpatients who had no history of addiction and who were administered opioids for the management of acute pain. He identified only four cases of drug dependence, and concluded that the development of addiction is an obscure event in medical patients with no history of addiction.

But opioid dependence, as I have defined the concept, is far from being a rare occurrence in general medicine. Countless pain patients use analgesics on a regular basis and are unwittingly caught in the paradoxical situation of experiencing pain as part of their ongoing opioid dependency. Still, the pharmaceutical companies continue to promise the public opioids that will free them from pain. It is now possible, for example, to ingest slow-release codeine capsules so that codeine is present in the nervous system on a 24-hour basis.

The use of opioids to control chronic pain is counterproductive to providing the individual with the necessary understanding and strategies required for recovery from the pain. The opening section of this chapter presented the distinction between drug efficacy and drug effectiveness. "Drug efficacy," in the case of analgesics, refers to how effective the medication is, relative to placebo or some other medication, in reducing pain. "Drug effectiveness" is a more encompassing term and refers to the degree to which the use of an analgesic allows the person to function in his/her natural environment and to carry out the normal activities of daily living. Thus an analgesic such as morphine or codeine can be efficacious if it lowers reported pain following ingestion but ineffective if the individual remains in bed all day following its use. It is beginning to be recognized that opioids are not effective in restoring an individual's sense of autonomy. With opioid use the patient remains dependent on medication as well as on the larger medical system for pain control:

> The person with chronic pain is limited not only by pain, but also by suffering which must be addressed before health is possible. Suffering implies threatened disintegration of the self and a loss of control and autonomy. It may be useful, therefore, to think of pain as being orthogonally related to autonomy. . . . Optimal pain management [requires a shift in both pain and autonomy whereby] pain is minimized and autonomy extended. There is, as yet, no evidence that opioid therapy will reliably create this shift in patients with chronic noncancer pain. We might expect improvement along the pain axis, but there are no data regarding the

autonomy axis. In fact, autonomy might be limited by the need to rely on medication. Chronic medical therapy fosters external rather than internal control, and so the locus of control is externalized. (Shug & Large, 1996, pp. 2–3)

Teaching patients how to utilize body awareness to manage pain becomes extremely difficult and often impossible if the patient remains dependent on opioid medication. Typically, the first signs of opioid withdrawal are interpreted as a sign of increasing pain and suffering, leading to fear that opioids must be used to relieve the pain. Having chronic patients grasp the idea that the pain and distress can be alleviated through somatic awareness strategies is best achieved if opioids and other analgesics are totally removed from the patient's treatment plan. However, there is no inherent reason why pain control through bodily awareness and medication cannot be used together. The difficulty is that patients who rely on analgesics do so exclusively and are too afraid to leave pain control to inner resources.

Health professionals face an enormous challenge in convincing chronic pain patients that there are alternatives to opioids in the management of their pain. Physicians can take a significant step in this direction by not believing that they must relieve all pain and suffering with medication. Walking through a geriatric rehabilitation hospital and listening to the pleas for more and/or stronger analgesic medication at times reminds one of an opium den. Physicians making rounds feel they have no choice other than to prescribe opioids as requested. Patients fully expect that their favorite analgesic will be provided on demand. It is far easier to give and take medication than it is to help patients find alternative strategies for managing a chronic pain problem.

Pain patient expectations regarding what can and cannot be achieved through opioids need to be tempered. After taking opioids for initial pain relief, they may eventually be forced to realize that the medication is worsening their pain. Simply discontinuing the medication will not be effective, unless there is a comprehensible strategy in place for managing pain without medication. Shug and Large (1995) recommend minimizing the problem by placing greater reliance on multidisciplinary interventions. A patient's physician does not have the resources to individually resolve the complex psychosocial and psychobiological issues contributing to chronic pain disorders. Multidisciplinary pain clinics have the advantage of being able to deal with pain management through psychosocial and biobehavioral approaches. Unfortunately, multidisciplinary pain clinics are not readily available to physicians and their patients and probably will become even less available with decreasing health care dollars.

Chronic pain patients need to take far more control of their pain condition. They need their physician to guide and assist their efforts, but the majority of change must come from psychobiological changes within themselves. Physicians can help by not promising to "fix" or "cure" conditions that they cannot possibly fix or cure and instead encourage the patient to learn to manage with less medication. Physicians can quite honestly and accurately state that in cases of long-standing chronic pain and opioid dependence, the withdrawal from opioids, if managed properly, will result in *less* rather than more pain. Patients who present to their physician with vague and poorly localized pain, with complaints of suffering, and with symptoms of throat and chest tightness should be advised, following the appropriate medical examinations, that their symptoms are in large part due to opioid use. Confidence in self-reliance comes very slowly and takes much hard work on the part of the patient and the therapist(s).

The widespread use of analgesic medications requires clearer recognition by patients and professionals alike of what can and cannot be achieved through medication use alone. The fact that chronic pain consists of pain, suffering, depression, and other affective states attests to the complex nature of the symptoms for which the drug is being used. The vast body of placebo research has taught us that the potential for mindful intentionality to effect therapeutic change is possible in every pain disorder. It is the very generality of the placebo effect that makes it mandatory that we learn to harness placebo power through somatic awareness interventions, even when using medications. In the pharmacological model of healing, knowledge is based exclusively on physician hypotheses about biochemical mechanisms and pharmacological interventions. Within the model, it does not matter what the patient believes, thinks, or feels. Within the holistic psychobiological framework, however, knowing, drug action, somatic awareness, and healing are all linked. A combination of self-regulatory beliefs and listening to the body are at the basis of therapeutic success, whether medication is used or not.

CHAPTER 4

Self-Regulation and Immunity

This chapter deals with somatic awareness and the immune system. The focus of discussion is the nature of bodily experiences that might be utilized to optimize the overall health of the immune system. In addition, I examine how individuals with immune system disease might best utilize somatic awareness to achieve disease management and/or remission. Considerable literature supports the hypothesis that diseases of the immune system are amenable to psychological influence and that the mind is capable of contributing to recovery from diseases that involve the immune system. People with diseases of the immune system recognize that, in addition to taking medication, they need to take care of themselves in terms of diet, exercise, sleep, and avoidance of stress. It is assumed that the collective practice of health behaviors might serve to strengthen or "boost" their immune system processes. Basic research continues to support this practice through demonstrations of links between psychological stress, emotional states, and immune system parameters.

Although the mind has no direct experiential link to the immune system, it is likely that feelings of bodily well-being are consistent with a healthy immune system. The same bodily information that is used to guide health with more specific physiological disorders such as headache and asthma can be used to direct recovery from immune system disease. Proprioceptive sensory information in particular is readily available but is often ignored or feared by the individuals with immune system illness. Long-term avoidance of bodily information may be a major predisposing factor for the onset of immune system illness. Since there is no research on the issue of somatic awareness and immune system disease, my discussion will be speculative. I build a case for somatic awareness and immunity by examining (1) the significance of nonspecific bodily tension; (2) the role of fatigue; and (3) the therapeutic value of qualitative adjustments in lifestyle. These factors are examined separately and in relation to arthritis, multiple sclerosis, and cancer. Although a different illness literature is used to examine each construct, it will be apparent that bodily tension, fatigue, and lifestyle are highly interrelated within each immune system illness.

THE NATURE OF PSYCHONEUROIMMUNOLOGY

Psychoneuroimmunology is the study of interactions between the mind, the nervous system, and the immune system. The term "interaction" is used to indicate that the relations between these various components are bidirectional. For example, the mind can influence the immune system and the immune system can influence the mind. The field of psychoneuroimmunology developed from the recognition that the immune system is not an autonomous system. The likelihood that somatic awareness might be used to facilitate immunoenhancement increased with the discovery that the function of the immune system depends, not only on local processes (production of T cells in a lymph node), but also on global alterations involving the entire organism (Maier, Watkins, & Fleshner, 1994). It is now established that major immune system organs such as the thymus, the bone marrow, the spleen, and the lymph nodes are innervated by the sympathetic nervous system. Immune system organs also contain catecholamine neurotransmitter receptors. Moreover, the terminals of the sympathetic nerve endings in these immune organs make contact with lymphocytes themselves—thus "the brain is physically connected to the immune system" (Maier et al., 1994, p. 1006). It is significant that the sympathetic nervous system, which is heavily involved in the mediation of emotions and feelings, is intricately involved with the immune system. If the brain is connected to the immune system, then so is the experiential mind.

Further support for the notion that experiential awareness of the body can play a role in immune system function is provided by the fact that the immune system and the neuroendocrine system are connected. Well-understood pathways between the mind and the neuroendocrine system are involved in the mediation of stress. The bodily effects of psychological and physical stress are associated with the release of steroid hormones, called glucocorticoids, from the outer portion of the adrenal gland (cortex). These events are initiated by the paraventricular nucleus of the hypothalamus, which secretes corticotropin-releasing hormone (CRH). CRH reaches the anterior lobe of the pituitary gland, effecting the synthesis and release of adrenocorticotropic hormone (ACTH) into the blood. ACTH, in turn, causes the release of glucocorticoids by the adrenal cortex. T and B lymphocytes are known to have receptors for glucocorticoids and other hormones. These lymphocytes also have catecholamine receptors that are sensitive to the release of norepinephrine and epinephrine from the inner portion of the adrenal gland (medulla). Thus anatomical pathways are in place for the brain–mind interface with immune system cells and organs. In the words of Maier et al. (1994), "Any psychological event that alters . . . neural and hormonal factors is capable of modulating immunity" (p. 1009). They use depression to illustrate their position. Depression is associated with the dysregulation of the pituitary-adrenal hormonal axis, and depressed individuals are known to have elevated glucocorticoid levels and to show evidence of immune system dysfunction.

A growing body of research links different psychosocial stressors to immune system alterations. This research is still preliminary and must be interpreted with caution when making extrapolations to relationships between stress and immune system function in the natural environment (Maier et al., 1994). Stress is generally associated with immunosuppression or what is called *downregulation* of the immune system. This conclusion is based on limited and isolated tests of immune system function, tests that may or may not reflect what takes place in the natural environment. The immune system changes that occur during the onset, development, and progression of a disease in a person's natural environment may be different than the immune system changes observed in limited laboratory situations.

Tests of the immune system are divided into *enumerative tests* and *functional tests*. An enumerative test or assay involves counting the numbers or percentages of different kinds of white blood cells (neutrophils, monocytes, lymphocytes) in the peripheral blood. Functional tests involve removing cells from the body and studying their function in the laboratory. For example, lymphocyte proliferation in a dish is a measure of immune system function designed to examine how effectively stimulated lymphocytes divide (i.e., proliferate). Lymphocytes are stimulated by incubating them with substances such as phytohemagglutinin (PHA), concanavalin A (Con A) and pokeweed mitogen (PWM). It is assumed that the more the lymphocytes (T cell or B cell) divide, the more effective the cells are functioning. Stress is associated with a decreased proliferative response of lymphocytes. A second functional test involves determining natural killer (NK) cell cytotoxic activity. NK cells serve a surveillance function within the immune system: they can detect and kill cancerous cells. The NK cell cytotoxic activity assay is an in vitro (outside the body) test in which NK cells are incubated with tumor cells. The immune cells are called "effector cells" because they affect the killing outcome and the tumor cells are called "targets." This assay is performed using a number of effector-to-target ratios (5:1, 10:1, 50:1, and 100:1). At higher ratios, more killing is expected to occur because of the greater number of effector cells that are available for every tumor target cell.

Research findings based on one or two isolated tests of the immune system represent an important beginning but must be interpreted with caution because they may or may not represent what actually takes place in an overall immune system response. The degree of proliferation of an individual's cells in response to mitogens might have no bearing on how the individual's immune system actually deals with the detection and clearing of specific antigens or the recognition and destruction of tumors and virally infected cells (Maier et al., 1994). In addition, the nature of a given immune response is likely to be highly individualistic and to vary with a number of parameters within the individual. Cohen and Herbert (1996) reviewed the relationship between mind and immunity with the aim of determining whether the literature supports the presence of a general link between psychological factors and immune system reactions. They also examined whether the literature supports a specific link between psychological factors and recovery from immune-system-mediated disease. Their review includes a series of studies that have examined the impact of psychological stress in naturalistic settings and in the laboratory on immune system parameters. The pioneer research in this area was carried out by Kiecolt-Glaser and Glaser (1988) in their investigations of the impact of medical school examinations on medical student's cellular immune function. In general, these studies reported decreased activity in a number of immune system parameters during and following the examination period. Similar conclusions suggestive of a link between emotional states and immunosuppression characterize the depression literature:

> A recent meta-analysis of over 40 studies shows that when compared to healthy controls, clinically depressed individuals have lowered proliferative response to PHA, Con A, and PWM; lowered NK activity; higher numbers of circulating white blood cells (primarily neutrophils and

monocytes); and lowered numbers of NK, B, T, helper T, and suppressor/
cytotoxic T cells. . . . Longitudinal data also suggest that when people
recover from depression, decreased NK activity is no longer evident. . . .
The relations between depression and immune outcomes are strongest in
both older and hospitalized samples. (Cohen & Herbert, 1996, p. 123)

The literature examining the relation between nonclinical dysthymic mood fluctuations and immunity is consistent with the clinical
depression findings: dysthymic mood is associated with decreased proliferative responses to mitogens and decreased NK activity, with the
effect sizes being about half those seen in clinical depression. Studies
are also beginning to report that fluctuations in positive and negative
mood across the same individuals are correlated with immune system
fluctuations. In the opening chapter, I noted that positive emotions are
associated with bodily feelings of lightness, warmth, and general well-
being. A study cited by Uchino, Cacioppo, and Kiecolt-Glaser (1996)
utilized a daily diary method to study the relations between positive
and negative mood states and antibody response to an orally ingested
antigen over 12 weeks. Antibody levels were higher on days when subjects reported high positive mood states and lower on days when they
reported high negative mood states. Perceived availability of social support has also been associated with enhanced immune function. Studies
have found enhanced immune function in persons reporting confiding
relationships and emotional support.

A few studies examining the association between social support
and HIV/AIDS progression have found that positive emotional support is associated with better immune system function (e.g., greater NK
cell lysis). However, given that AIDS is an extremely complex disease, it
is not surprising that research in this area is difficult both to conduct
and to interpret. For example, studies that have examined the relationship between social support and HIV progression in gay men have produced conflicting results, with some studies reporting a positive relationship and others not (Uchino et al., 1996). Still, there is reason for
cautious optimism: recent studies suggest that the progression of HIV
might be delayed through social support. In a prospective study across
a 5-year period, Theorell et al. (1995) found that the availability of
social and emotional support predicted subsequent changes in CD4
counts in a representative sample of men with HIV. CD4 T lymphocytes are immune system cells whose levels decrease over the course of
HIV infection. The results revealed that high and low social support
groups did not differ in CD4 counts during the early years of the study.
However, the prediction of CD4 counts as a function of social support
was evident during years 4 and 5 of the study. For instance, during year

5 of the study, individuals high in social support showed a –37% change in CD4 counts, whereas individuals low in social support showed a –64% change in CD4 counts.

Intimate relationships are a powerful form of social support and likely also a powerful source of immunoenhancement. Intuitively, we recognize that intimate interactions foster a natural sense of body comfort and inner peace in both members of the relationship. Intimacy itself is a multidimensional feeling state and includes guidance, alliances, reassurances of worth, social integration, attachment, and opportunities for nurturance (Baron, Cutrona, Hicklin, Russell, & Lubaroff, 1990). The loss of an intimate relationship through death is one of the most stressful of all life experiences. In a longitudinal study of bereavement, Kemeny et al. (1995) examined whether immune changes indicative of HIV progression occurred in gay men whose intimate partners had died of AIDS during the past year. The data were obtained from participants enrolled in the Multicenter AIDS Cohort Study (MACS) which began in Los Angeles in 1984 and involved 1,637 gay and bisexual men. Participants in the sample are examined at regular 6-month intervals for signs and symptoms of AIDS. A blood sample is obtained at each interval and the fresh blood is analyzed for a number of lymphocyte subsets, including CD4 T cells and NK cells. The investigators also examine the frozen sera for the presence of immune activation by measuring neopterin levels as well as proliferative response to PHA.

This report is based on two blood samples for each bereaved partner, one drawn before the death of the partner and one drawn within 13 months after the death of the partner. For each nonbereaved control subject, two blood samples were obtained over an equivalent time period. The results were suggestive of changes in the immune systems of the bereaved subjects: there was a significant increase in neopterin levels and a significant decrease in the proliferative response to PHA after the death of a partner. These significant changes were not matched by similar changes in the nonbereaved individuals. No significant differences were found for CD4 T cell levels. According to the authors, the increase in neopterin in the bereaved individuals is a strong predictor of the development of AIDS:

> Neopterin is produced by activated monocytes in response to cytokine signals, such as γ-interferon. In a variety of epidemiologic studies, including those conducted in our laboratory, an increase in serum neopterin levels in the blood of HIV-seropositive men has been shown to be a strong predictor of the development of AIDS, independent of the number of CD4 T cells. These reports indicate that neopterin values of 20 (nmol/l) or above

conferred a greater risk of developing AIDS than values below 15. The average increase from 13 to 20 nmol/l after the death of their partners placed the bereaved group in this higher risk range. (p. 552)

The decrease in the proliferative response to the mitogen PHA of the bereaved men following the death of their partners has been observed in other studies of spousal bereavement. It is interesting that no immune changes were found after the death of an intimate partner in the HIV-seronegative men observed in the study. The researchers speculate that the death of a partner to HIV-related disease may be much more of a profound loss for men who know that they themselves are HIV-positive.

A second study by this group (Cole, Kemeny, & Taylor, 1997) demonstrated how the awareness of bodily self is likely to be heavily influenced by how one feels he or she is viewed by members of society. It is difficult to maintain an internal sense of bodily equilibrium in the face of perceived rejection, ostracism, and fear of assault. Gay men live with the threat of homophobic social rejection. Cole et al. developed the hypothesis that gay men infected with HIV would be more vulnerable to disease progression if they were also sensitive to social rejection. As part of the MACS, they presented additional data on HIV-seropositive gay men who were observed at 6-month intervals over the 9-year study period. In this study they asked whether the HIV-seropositive men who were high on social rejection would also be more vulnerable to disease progression than seropositive gay men who were not high on social rejection. Social rejection was measured by a questionnaire that asked the men to indicate their degree of discomfort in a variety of social situations such as going out in public with a group of gay men, going to a straight party alone, and having relatives in their home with their partners present.

The results provided solid support for the harmful effects of perceived social rejection: the subjects who scored high on the rejection-sensitivity questionnaire showed definite signs of more rapid disease progression in terms of (1) shorter times to critically low CD4 T lymphocyte levels, (2) shorter times to AIDS diagnosis, and (3) shorter times to HIV-related mortality. To explain their findings, Cole et al. draw from the developmental research of Kagan (1994), who found that individuals who exhibit extreme shyness or inhibited social characteristics, including reduced emotional expressiveness, heightened sensitivity to the presence of others, and a tendency to withdraw in the presence of others, may also exhibit heightened sympathetic nervous system activity. I have already observed that variations in sympathetic nervous system activity can influence immune system function. More immediate to somatic awareness, sensitivity to social rejection can generate bodily feelings of vague discomfort and tension. Thus sensitivity to rejection needs to be kept in mind when working with individuals with chronic disease. Sensitivity to rejection cannot be allowed to counteract the potential healing benefits of somatic awareness.

It is obvious that a caring social and family environment promotes the ability to care for oneself. Without support, the afflicted individual has greater difficulty identifying the inner healing resources needed to lessen the risk of disease progression. It is difficult to imagine how HIV-infected individuals can be expected to establish and maintain a state of inner bodily awareness if they are marginalized and stigmatized by the larger society. HIV is a formidable illness, and no one should be required to deal with it alone. This is especially true for children infected with HIV. Children born with HIV live on average 9.4 years and are moderately symptomatic for more than half their expected lives. These children are attending day care programs and schools and require special understanding and care. We need to identify new strategies whereby children, families of children, peers, and educators work together to determine ways in which somatic awareness might be used to minimize HIV-disease progression.

Although the majority of research has examined the influence of psychological processes on the immune system, it is also possible that the state of the immune system might influence a person's psychological state. Preliminary research with animals has found detectable changes in the brain following activation of the immune system by an antigen (Maier et al., 1994). One hypothesis holds that the link from the immune system to the brain involves cytokines, soluble proteins released by the immune system. Cytokines such as interleukin-1 (IL-1) are believed to be capable of generating peripheral physiological responses similar to those that occur during a response to stress. Maier et al. demonstrated that the release of cytokines might activate neural circuits involved in pain. In preliminary research, they found that the induction of illness and immune activation in rats was accompanied by hyperalgesia or increased sensitivity to painful stimuli, which they hypothesized resulted from IL-1 activation of hyperalgesia circuitry in the brain and spinal cord. Maier has also demonstrated that immune system messengers such as IL-1 might activate clumps of nerve cells called "paraganglia," which in turn activate the vagus to relay information to the brain (Pennisi, 1997). Similar immunological messengers might send information to the brain and contribute to mood swings as well as to bodily feelings associated with poor health such as heightened pain sensitivity and feelings of chronic fatigue.

The literature has documented that the brain can shape the

immune response. It remains to be proven whether immunosuppression, mind-induced or otherwise, is responsible for disease onset. The demonstrated relationships between psychological variables and immune system function have been small, and little is known concerning the health consequences of such changes. Cohen and Herbert (1996) concluded that firm conclusions regarding psychological causality, immunosuppression, and disease onset are not possible at this time. With respect to colds and influenza, for example, they observed correlations between measures of psychological stress and symptom onset. At the same time, changes in various measures of white blood cells failed to predict the onset of cold and flu symptoms. Could it be, they ask, that people under stress simply seek out the companionship of others and consequently expose themselves to infectious agents?

In spite of the struggling inherent with a new model, the psychoimmunological approach continues to gain acceptance and momentum. There is sufficient research demonstrating that psychological factors influence the immune system and that complex interactions take place between the different systems involving mind, brain, and body. More and more scientists are accepting the notion that maintaining and/or restoring health requires getting beyond the individual level of immune cells, neurons, and behavior. The field of psychoneuroimmunology is leading to the reemergence of ideas about how medical science needs to reverse its thinking regarding the bacterial, viral, and other agents that are suspected of disrupting immune system function.

THE OPTIMUM STATE OF EMBODIMENT

The idea that the overall psychobiological health of the person is crucial to disease prevention and recovery is gaining momentum. Louis Pasteur (1822–1895) is credited with the prophetic statement, *"Bernard avait raison. Le germe n'est pas rien, c'est le terrain qui est tout"* ("Bernard was right. The germ is nothing, the soil is everything"; Ornstein & Sobel, 1987). Pincus (1996), for example, expressed the opinion that the state of the organism is more important than the infectious agent in understanding disease outcome:

> The principles of the germ theory were coded in a set of criteria known as Koch's Postulates, developed by Robert Koch [1843–1910], who identified the tubercle bacillus in patients with tuberculosis, the most feared disease in the nineteenth century. The aim of the Postulates was to set standards that had to be met to establish an association between a specific infectious

agent and a disease. The Postulates stipulate that the infectious agent should be identified in each individual with a specific disease, that it should be isolated in a pure culture and then produce a similar disease in experimental animals, and that the agent should then be recovered from diseased animals. . . .

The critical point is that the Postulates address only the infectious *agent*. They ignore entirely the *host*, including the host's genetic background, age, physiological and psychological status; the presence in the host of other diseases; and the host's environment, including housing, sanitation, and other conditions that may protect from or predispose to disease. All infectious agents and hosts interact in a milieu of internal host defenses and regulatory mechanisms, and external physical and socioeconomic environmental conditions. There is no doubt that certain individuals have host defenses that reduce the likelihood of a deleterious outcome from an infectious agent or even prevent infection from that agent. After all, if some members of a species did not have the internal resources to defend themselves against an infectious agent, the agent theoretically would eradicate the species (and thereby, if it were a virus, itself). Even the Ebola and human immunodeficiency virus are met by host defense mechanisms in certain individuals. (pp. 64–65)

Now that it is understood that, at both the anatomical and the functional levels, there are connections between the brain, the autonomic nervous system, and the immune system, the question is whether the human mind has the capability to capture the adaptive nature of the immune system through conscious experience. The issue might be phrased as determining "how ephemeral phenomena of the psyche can be translated into a healing immunologic process" (Lloyd, 1996, p. 5). In other words, is there an optimum state of mind associated with healing from immune system disease? Lloyd speculated that part of the answer might be found in a link between the psychological self and the immune system, for it is the self that defines the core of an individual. A harmonious self might embody a harmonious or healthy immune system:

Thus, the Russian embryologist and immunologist, Elie Metchnikoff, writing in the late nineteenth century, extrapolated from his studies of the workings of the phagocyte (a white blood cell capable of ingesting extracellular, particulate matter) to envision the living organism as "intrinsically disharmonious and striving for harmony." . . . Given his rigorous, unsentimental grasp of the reality of the organism, whether vertebrate or invertebrate, Metchnikoff saw direct affinity between the protective imperatives of immunity in the most primitive of organisms and evolution of the self in the human organism. (p. 10)

Other theorists have suggested that psychological concepts such as meaning, coherence, connectedness, and spiritual purpose need to be incorporated into theoretical understandings of a healthy immune system. All such concepts are valid to the extent that their adoption leads to activation of the psychobiological processes influencing immune system health. Somatic awareness represents an experiential construct for organizing, integrating, and facilitating the various factors in a therapeutic fashion. Without such integration, the individual runs the risk of not enhancing the strength of his/her immune system through the adoption of a particular belief or behavioral strategy.

Virtually all major treatment centers for illnesses involving the immune system provide patients with a variety of self-regulatory therapies. Visualization, relaxation, prayer, humor, biofeedback, massage, and group therapy represent some of the more popular self-regulatory strategies in use today. Patients using any of these techniques would presumably benefit from a framework for understanding what they are supposed to experience in order to maximize their chances of recovery. For example, what is the healing process behind visualizing white blood cells destroying cancer cells or making oneself laugh once a day? How does relaxation or attending group therapy sessions lead to disease remission? How does a mantra or a prayer heal? There has to be some identifiable psychobiological process that mediates between the act of visualizing, praying, or engaging in other self-regulatory strategies and the response of the immune system. Even more critical is providing the patient with an understanding of what to do in the time *between* the practice of specific techniques. Patients need an experiential means for integrating the practice of one or more of these techniques into their daily consciousness. What does one do, for example, between times of visualization or prayer? There has to be a way to experience wellness on a continuous basis.

The need for an integrative concept to synthesize the alternative strategies currently in use with immune diseases is obvious. There also has to be some way for the individual to experience this inner process. Otherwise he/she will not know whether it is being used to the best extent possible. I offer somatic awareness as the experiential link between mind and the immune system. I propose that the same process postulated to underlie placebo effects can boost the body's immune system. By utilizing somatic awareness as a means of enhancing the healing power of his/her immune system, the individual can avail him/herself of an experiential guide to selecting which health behaviors are most likely to be of value and how these behaviors may need to be fashioned on a moment-to-moment basis. To illustrate, one individual may through prayer and spiritual conviction find that his/ her disease enters remission, and consequently may believe that his/ her prayers were answered. The next individual with the same disease may engage in exactly the same religious practice and experience no improvement in his/her disease condition. The latter individual may feel emotionally betrayed. Personal beliefs, feelings, and attitudes are a necessary part of the puzzle to immunoregulation, but these psychological events must bring about changes in psychoneuroimmunological processes that facilitate health. We need a better understanding of how to activate these processes, regardless of our particular faith or self-help preferences.

Benson (1996) provided an example of how a patient successfully combined her religious beliefs, interpersonal connectedness, and bodily awareness to manage anxiety triggered by the threat of cancer. The "relaxation response" is Benson's recommended way to calm the body and achieve somatic awareness. He states that there are only two steps to eliciting the response: (1) repeating a word, sound, phrase, or muscular activity; and (2) passively disregarding everyday thoughts that come to mind. The patient in question decided to incorporate a religious phrase into her practice of the relaxation response:

> Since I encourage people to pick a focus that pleases them, she adopted a Spanish blessing, "*Jesu Christo ayudame, amparame y curame,*" which means "Jesus Christ, help me, protect me, and cure me." Her mother said a similar blessing to her and her siblings as children before they left for school each day. And over the course of months in which she used this familiar prayer to elicit the relaxation response, Ms. Baquero began to feel liberated from the worry and strain that had bothered her incessantly before. "I started to feel better. I started looking at people and life in a different way. I put less pressure on myself," she says.
>
> Surely, Ms. Baquero was experiencing the wonderful physiological solace of the relaxation response, the opposite effect of the edgy, adrenaline rush we experience in the stress-induced fight-or-flight response. But she also spoke of a more emotional comfort, which the symbolism and meaning of her mother's blessing inspired. The emotional and spiritual balm seemed to affect her as much as the chemical and physical changes that occur during the relaxation response. Not only was her body soothing itself but Ms. Baquero seemed to be reclaiming her identity—the essence of which was called into question when the threat of cancer was introduced to her. Each time she invoked this powerful prayer, she recalled her mother's faith in God's protection, and the faith instilled in her as a child. By introducing this tender comfort into her daily experience, she began to regain confidence both in her body and in herself to face the twists and turns of life. (p. 19)

This is an excellent case study of a patient who was able to integrate meaning, spirituality, and bodily awareness to improve the quality of her life and her overall health.

Ms. Baquero had her faith to guide her in self-discovery. The question remains whether somatic awareness can be as powerful without such faith. Benson (1996) takes the position that whether God created us or whether we created God to cover up the meaninglessness of existence, the fact is that humans are *wired for God*:

> In what I know must seem coldly analytical to those who fervently believe in God, faith is a win–win situation when it comes to our bodies. Believing that God exists, or simply believing that God is food for a brain that craves it, allows humans to reap rewards in both improved health and in greater personal fulfillment. Faith is good for us, whether you believe that God planted these genes within us or whether you believe that humans created the idea of God to nourish a body yearning to survive. (p. 211)

Humans may be "wired" for spirituality, as Benson states, but there is not necessarily a direct connection between believing in a greater power than ourselves and improved health. Ms. Baquero's faith provided her with a powerful means of soothing herself and reclaiming her identity. However, bodily well-being can be achieved in any number of ways. Humans may have an even stronger wiring for somatic awareness since it is possible to utilize the healing effects of bodily experiences regardless of one's secular or religious worldview. Somatic awareness is the ultimate experiential heuristic in guiding individuals toward internal forces that can maximize the healing forces of the body. At the same time, it is important to integrate somatic awareness with other aspects of an individual's psychological, physiological, and interpersonal day-to-day life.

The need to examine somatic awareness and immunity from both a psychobiological and a systemic perspective is apparent in the following discussion of several immune system illnesses. A case is made for nonspecific bodily tension and fatigue as significant risk factors for arthritis and multiple sclerosis and, by implication, for cancer as well. The issue is whether individuals with diseases of the immune system can, through the development of somatic awareness, achieve significant reductions in chronic tension and fatigue and thereby arrest and/or reverse underlying disease processes. A related issue is whether they also need to make changes within themselves with respect to psychological and interpersonal issues. Must they, in developing a sense of bodily well-being, change the way they think about their lives and the people they care most about?

NONSPECIFIC BODILY TENSION IN ARTHRITIS

Rheumatoid arthritis is an autoimmune disease marked by chronic inflammation of joints of the body. An autoimmune disease is characterized by the body attacking its own cells and organs. The immune system produces antibodies that attack its own tissue, and T lymphocytes fail to discern self from nonself and therefore attack healthy body tissue. It is unknown what factors set the antibody process into action. One hypothesis advanced for rheumatoid arthritis and other autoimmune conditions is that the disease process is triggered, in genetically susceptible individuals, by bacterial antigens or viruses, although neither has yet been identified.

Most individuals afflicted with rheumatoid arthritis exhibit a chronic fluctuating course of disease that, if left untreated, results in progressive joint destruction, deformity, disability, and premature death (American College of Rheumatology, 1996). It is the most prevalent chronic condition in women in the United States. It is estimated that by the year 2020 the percentage of affected women will exceed a quarter of the population of women aged 15 years and older (Callahan, 1996). In addition to being the most prevalent chronic condition in women, arthritis is also the leading cause of physical limitations in women. Arthritis is a significant women's health issue and deserves much more attention in this regard. The number-one risk factor for most rheumatic diseases, including fibromyalgia and osteoarthritis, is being a woman (Hannan, 1996). Although hormonal explanations are usually offered to explain the higher incidence of arthritis in women, one cannot help but notice that the gender that historically has had the least opportunity to self-soothe is the one most vulnerable to the disease.

Studies consistently show that women experience relatively high psychological demands in terms of paid work and family work, with time constraints being a very frequently cited problem. Family demands may be more important than work demands in this regard. It is ironic that women, who epitomize caring, are often not allowed the time necessary to care for themselves. In genetically susceptible women, the lack of opportunity for self-soothing may be a major precursor of rheumatoid arthritis.

Rheumatoid arthritis is characterized by a symmetric pattern of joint inflammation involving the wrists, bones of the hand, fingers, feet, toes, elbows, shoulders, hips, knees, and ankles (Miller-Blair & Robbins, 1993). Swelling and pain in one or more joints for a period of at least 6 weeks are required for a diagnosis of rheumatoid arthritis (Lorig & Fries, 1995). The inflammation is accompanied by pain and stiffness of the involved joints, in particular by a phenomenon known as "gelling" in which the joints are stiff after a period of rest, especially in the morning.

> Usually, there are general problems such as muscle aches, fatigue, muscle stiffness (particularly in the morning), and even a low fever. Morning stiffness is often considered a hallmark of RA [rheumatoid arthritis] and is sometimes termed the *gel phenomenon*. After a rest period or even after just sitting motionless for a few minutes, the whole body feels stiff and is difficult to move. After a period of loosening up, motion becomes easier and less painful. (Lorig & Fries, 1995, p. 9)

In our bodies, cartilage caps the end of each bone and serves to keep the bones from rubbing together. The synovium is a membrane-lined sac that covers the joint and produces synovial fluid, a clear lubricating fluid that serves to "grease" the joint. During inflammation of the joint (termed "synovitis") damage to the small blood vessels allows monocytes in the synovial membrane to accumulate around the deranged capillaries. T lymphocytes then initiate a series of changes in cytokines, B cell proliferation, and antibody production. Together these events lead to inflammation and the production of invasive granulation tissue called "pannus." Joint destruction begins in bare areas of bone not covered with cartilage and results from invasive growth by the pannus and from exposure to inflammatory by-products.

Fibromyalgia, a common chronic pain disorder, is considered a variant of rheumatoid arthritis. Fibromyalgia patients describe their pain as annoying, nagging, troublesome, and exhausting. Fibromyalgia is a *soft tissue* rheumatic disorder. It begins between the ages of 35 and 50 years and affects women eight to nine times more frequently than men (Merskey, 1996). Prior to 1980 fibromyalgia was not a frequent diagnosis but fibromyalgia is now the second most frequent referral to rheumatologists. The cardinal symptom of fibromyalgia is widespread body pain. For a diagnosis to be made, the pain must be present in a diffuse fashion, involving some part of the body on the left and right sides both above and below the waist. The pain usually begins locally and begins to spread following the segmental organization of the spinal cord. Patients also need to be tender at 11 of 18 defined tender points. In general, these tender points occur at muscle tendon junctions. An interesting observation is that fibromyalgia patients were less able to relax their muscles in the short pauses between isokinetic muscle contractions and had increased muscle fatigability compared with healthy controls (Bennett, 1996). This observation may also reflect poorly on their ability to relax.

The ultimate goal of therapy in rheumatoid arthritis is to achieve a remission or reduction of the symptoms of active inflammatory joint pain, morning stiffness, fatigue, synovitis, and joint damage. Complete remission is seldom achieved; thus management goals are directed toward reducing disease activity, alleviating pain, and maintaining the activities of daily living. Drug treatment for rheumatoid arthritis usually involves, at least initially, the use of nonsteroidal anti-inflammatory drugs (NSAIDs) to reduce joint pain and swelling and improve function. NSAIDs have analgesic and anti-inflammatory properties but do not influence the course of the disease or prevent joint destruction. There is a class of drugs, called disease-modifying antirheumatic drugs (DMARDs), that have the potential to reduce or prevent joint damage. These drugs include oral gold, hydroxychloroquine, and methotrexate. Unfortunately, all of these drugs have a potential toxicity (American College of Rheumatology, 1996).

Given the seriousness of rheumatoid arthritis and the aggressive drug treatment that it often requires, it may seem that there is little opportunity for self-regulatory strategies based on somatic awareness to have a significant impact on the disease. The problem of using somatic awareness with this autoimmune condition, as with other autoimmune conditions, is that the afflicted individuals believe strongly that the disease and its symptoms occur outside their psychological influence. Moreover, their preferred coping style is to ignore their body as much as possible, usually because it is swollen and painful, and in severe cases because it is disfigured.

Rheumatoid arthritis is, to a very significant extent, a musculoskeletal disease (Afable & Ettinger, 1993). Pain and fatigue, the most common symptoms of musculoskeletal disease, are generally experienced as evidence that the arthritic condition is worsening. It is quite possible that the musculoskeletal disease and symptoms of rheumatoid arthritis have their origins in a musculoskeletal envelope of tension. There is no direct evidence for this hypothesis and no way of measuring the hypothesized envelope of pervasive muscle tension. The existence of such tension, however, is consistent with the lifestyles and personality attributes of many arthritics who suffer from pain. Diffuse pain is usually attributed directly to the underlying inflammatory process and not to psychobiological variables associated with musculoskeletal tension.

Pervasive muscle tension likely contributes to all autoimmune conditions associated with chronic fatigue and pain. The International Association for the Study of Pain (1986) defined a condition called "myofascial pain syndrome" as diffuse aching musculoskeletal pain associated with multiple discrete tender points and stiffness. The pain is widespread, is perceived as deep, and is usually referred to muscle or bony prominences. There is day-to-day fluctuation in pain intensity as well as pain shifting from one body location to another. Stiffness is common and is especially bad in the mornings. Rosomoff, Fishbain, Goldberg, Santana, and Rosomoff (1989) carried out physical examinations of a large sample of patients who had chronic neck and back pain. Chronic pain was defined as pain with a duration of 6 months or longer. Through palpation, they identified tender/trigger points in 98.4% of the sample, followed by 68.6% reporting decreased range of motion. Similar symptoms are often interpreted as indicative of some rheumatic disease process such as fibromyalgia, but it makes good clinical sense to view their origins as more psychobiological and musculoskeletal in nature. Tender/trigger points are, after all, the same as tender muscle motor points. Rosomoff et al. excluded from their analysis patients with definite evidence of physical and/or degenerative disease. However, they noted that even after "successful" surgical treatment for nerve root compression and herniated disks, the pain often persists. The prolongation of the pain condition reflects, in their view, the failure to resolve the musculoskeletal abnormalities that produce and maintain the painful state. In my view, patients with persistent pain have yet to experience how somatic awareness can be utilized to manage their symptom.

If pervasive muscle tension is a major contributor to rheumatoid arthritis, the question remains as to the origins of this tension. The answer to this question, as I stated earlier, must have some bearing on why arthritis afflicts three times as many women as men. Rheumatoid arthritis was one of the original "Chicago Seven" psychosomatic diseases cited by Franz Alexander (1950) within his psychoanalytic specificity theory. He described the mental traits of individuals susceptible to arthritis as emotionally controlling, demanding, and domineering. They are also rejecting of feminine attributes, competitive with men, and driven to serve other people. Although such broad descriptions have not been supported through group research, there is a clinical sense that emotional suppression and lifelong stress may characterize individuals with rheumatoid arthritis. Consider the following psychological description of patients with chronic fatigue symptoms. The description applies equally well to many arthritic patients:

> CFS [chronic fatigue syndrome] sufferers in the U.S. . . . were leading lives of intense activity and involvement before their illness began. Believing in the value of hard work, those who were employed devoted 60, 70, or even 80 hours a week to their jobs. Employment was combined with major responsibilities in other domains, such as child-rearing, graduate study, and/or attending to the needs of an aging or ill parent. A desire for

accomplishment and success, underwritten by exacting standards for personal performance, impelled these individuals always to try harder, go further, in an attempt to meet the expectations they had set for themselves at work, at home, and at school. The result was an overextended, overcommitted lifestyle that left them feeling breathless—fragmented by competing demands, straining toward achievement and "perfection," constantly pressed for time. . . .

Also evident in sufferers' accounts of their lives before CFS is an inclination toward self-effacement—a tendency to place the interests of others ahead of their own concerns. Interviewees spoke of "taking care of other people," of "trying to make other people happy" to the point of neglecting, perhaps harming themselves. . . . Unable to resist the responsibilities that feeling "needed" entailed, they reported "giving too much" to families, employers and friends, then "having too little" left over for themselves.

Finally, the life histories recounted by study participants contain evidence of considerable distress. . . . Negative life events in the form of serious injury, divorce, job loss, and/or death of a family member or close friend were reported prior to CFS onset by a large proportion of the sample. Chronic difficulties such as serious illness in the immediate family, a troubled or failing marriage, and/or persistent problems at work were also described by many. Approximately half of the subjects represented their childhoods in terms that suggested the presence of significant depression or anxiety, alcohol or other drug abuse, and/or physical violence in parents or other close family members. Physical, sexual, or verbal abuse; low self-esteem; and chronic tension or fighting in the family were other recurring childhood themes. (Ware & Kleinman, 1992, pp. 551–552)

These individuals were highly responsible individuals who paid attention to everyone but themselves. They were likely completely unaware of the negative impact their lifestyles were having on their own bodily functioning. Symptoms of tension and pain, when they could no longer be ignored, were often attributed to mysterious viral agents. Significantly, those who recovered from the illness were those who were able to take stock of their lives and reevaluate their priorities—generally leading to increased recognition of their own psychological and somatic needs. Those who successfully recovered were able to "let go" of their previous lifestyle. They recognized that a life of hard work and a need for success were overvalued and destructive of their psychological and somatic well-being.

The postulated link between somatic awareness and a healthy immune system is speculative and difficult to advance at the research level. However, the idea is consistent with clinical observations that have been made throughout the ages. Astute clinicians have long suspected that certain personality and emotional styles characterize individuals with immune disease. A modern formulation of these attributes is the Type C coping style, as presented by Temoshok (1990). The Type C coping style is described as "being 'nice,' stoic or self-sacrificing, cooperative and appeasing, unassertive, patient, compliant with external authorities, and unexpressive of negative emotions, particularly anger" (p. 209). Temoshok would be the first to argue that it would be a gross oversimplification to imply that such attributes, in isolation, cause disease. However, she believes that the Type C coping pattern may be one factor in the development of an immune illness. Also, the same attributes may influence the course of an immune illness should such an illness develop.

The personality/emotional attributes characteristic of Type C coping, with their heavy orientation toward pleasing and not offending others, tend to minimize internal somatic awareness and to maintain musculoskeletal tension. These attributes often lead the individual to avoid personal emotional and bodily feelings in order to meet perceived external expectations and responsibilities. Why are these individuals low in somatic awareness? It appears, as suggested in the discussion of hypnotizability and somatization, that denial of emotional feelings goes hand in hand with denial of physical feelings. Given that emotions themselves consist of psychological and physiological properties, it would follow that denial of emotional feelings would lead to lack of awareness at all levels.

Individuals with highly controlled emotional coping styles in combination with a physical symptom focus are not easy to teach somatic awareness. In part, they are victims of the cultural view that taking care of themselves or self-soothing is a sign of personal weakness. If they have lived difficult lives, they may have worked, out of necessity, very hard at ignoring their bodies in order to stay in control of themselves and their life circumstance. The prospect of attaining a state of bodily well-being through somatic awareness may be synonymous in their experience with losing control of both their body and their mind.

Patients with arthritic disease often require considerable therapy before they are willing to entertain the notion of working with bodily experience to restore health. This is the case even though they often recognize that stress is associated with flare-ups of their symptoms. Because of their controlling style, they may also be especially sensitive to interpersonal conflict. Given that these are very independent and strong-willed individuals, they might have a difficult time showing "weakness" in the presence of friends and caregivers. In addition, their arthritic condition, especially if severe and associated with disfigurement and disability, might have initiated a degree of clinical depression that also needs treatment. The demoralization and feelings of helplessness that accompany depression may need to be dealt with initially in order to provide the patient with the necessary personal resources to deal with the disease processes.

The professional treatment of arthritis has evolved beyond medication. There are a number of excellent programs for guiding the management of rheumatoid arthritis. The best known of the arthritic self-management programs comes from Lorig and associates (Lorig & Fries, 1995). Their program provides suggestions and strategies for dealing with all aspects of the illness, including activities of daily living (e.g., dressing, bathing, cooking, working), strategies for maintaining strength and flexibility, diet, medication, and pain management. Cognitive therapy is often used to tackle helplessness beliefs and to improve self-efficacy.

Although arthritis care is now comprehensive, programs would benefit from explicit somatic awareness development. Psychological studies of rheumatoid arthritis patients generally ignore the possibility that psychobiological processes contribute to rheumatoid arthritis and may also be used to slow or even reverse the disease process. Instead the research adopts the illness behavior perspective, which separates psychological and disease variables. Rather than postulate psychobiological factors that might lead to the remission of the disease, these studies deal with individual differences in how afflicted individuals cope with the disease. Thus, it is assumed that the disease is caused by some unknown viral agent and once present the psychological characteristics of the individual determine how debilitating the disease becomes in terms of quality-of-life indices.

Illness behavior models are important for providing formulations of how differences in coping styles of individuals with the same disease influence associated disability levels and quality of life. "Disability" is defined as a limitation of function that compromises an individual's ability to perform an activity with the range considered normal (Bennett, 1996). Devins, Edworthy, Guthrie, and Martin (1992), for example, presented an illness behavior model based on the concept of *illness intrusiveness*. The first stage in their descriptive model is characterized by the onset of inflammatory changes in the joints, which lead to further biochemical changes, resulting in damage to the cartilage, bone, ligaments, and tendons surrounding each joint. These anatomical changes are accompanied by reductions in range of motion and decreased strength associated with specific functional deficits (e.g., the ability to pinch the fingers). Eventually the development of specific physical limitations leads to more general lifestyle disruptions and interference with activities and interests, or what they call "illness intrusiveness." Illness intrusiveness then results in somatic distress and decreased psychological well-being, which in turn worsen the pain and other symptoms present.

The illness intrusiveness concept is similar in meaning to more general models of illness behavior. These models all deal with how one copes with disease rather than with how one influences underlying disease processes. Remaining active is generally viewed as more positive than taking to bed and restricting social activities. Coping attempts are primarily determined by appraisals of the disease and its associated limitations. "For instance, interpreting disease as a permanent harm that one is helpless to influence promotes passive coping and is likely to result in depressive symptoms, whereas interpreting disease as a challenge to be overcome promotes more active coping" (Smith & Wallston, 1992, p. 152). A self-report instrument that is used extensively with rheumatic disease patients is the Coping Strategies Questionnaire (CSQ; Keefe et al., 1991). Research has found that individuals who employ positive coping self-statements (e.g., "I tell myself to be brave and carry on despite the pain"), who ignore painful sensations (e.g., "I tell myself it doesn't hurt"), and who maintain high activity (e.g., "I do something active, like household chores or projects") also exhibit higher levels of psychological function. At the same time, however, there is no evidence that differences in cognitive coping styles influence the underlying disease process itself (Burckhardt, Clark, O'Reilly, & Bennett, 1997).

Other data support the notion that illness behavior and disease mechanisms are independent events. Salaffi, Cavalieri, Nolli, and Ferraccioli (1991) examined the relationship between the degree of knee damage present in women with osteoarthritis, subjective pain experienced, and level of reported disability. Knee damage was determined from radiographs that measured a number of physical variables, including joint erosion, narrowing of joint space, calcification, malalignment, and swelling. The radiological variables were graded to provide a single "knee score." Also measured were the subjects' ratings of pain associated with the knee arthritis, self-reported anxiety and depression, and perceived functional impairment. "Functional impairment" referred to the degree to which subjects felt that their arthritis impaired their physical activity, household activities, social activity, and activities of daily living. There was no statistical relationship between the radiological index of knee damage and patient-perceived functional disability. The amount of objectively determined knee arthritis was not predictive of perceived disability due to arthritis. Self-reports of pain, anxiety, and depression were also not related to the radiological findings. Psychological variables of anxiety and depression, however, did predict the amount of pain experienced. Pain is the major symptom of knee arthritis, and it was better predicted by psychological variables than by anatomical damage as determined by radiological assessment.

Studies of illness behavior are a double-edged sword in terms of holistic models of chronic disease development and management. Illness behavior observations demonstrate how psychological characteristics of the individual, for example, anxiety and depression, influence coping with underlying disease processes. Illness behavior models, however, have the unfortunate effect of separating mind and body disease processes. In the above example, it was assumed that the extent of knee damage and the psychological reaction to knee damage are independent events. Illness behavior explanations tend to support a level of separation or dualism between the disease process itself and how one copes with the disease.

The suggested limitation of illness behavior models in dealing with arthritis at the psychobiological level is supported by some outcome findings of Lorig et al. (1989) regarding their own program. They examined what individuals actually learn when they successfully complete their arthritic self-management program. Lorig et al.'s program depends heavily on minimizing illness behaviors and practicing health behaviors related to exercise and relaxation. They measure improvement in health status in terms of changes in self-reported daily disability, pain, and depression. Interestingly, they found that individuals who had received instruction in the pathophysiology of arthritis, individual exercise and relaxation, joint protection methods, and techniques for solving arthritis-related problems did no better in managing their pain and disability than a control group who received no such intervention. This finding occurred in spite of the fact that the treatment group, relative to the controls, exhibited more arthritis self-management knowledge and engaged in more self-management activities such as walking, swimming, cycling, relaxation, and specific arthritic exercises. This finding is important for our discussion of somatic awareness. The treated patients were engaging in healthy behaviors but not feeling improved in terms of experienced disability, pain, and depression. I suspect that the treated patients had learned to reduce their illness behaviors but they had not learned how to alter the somatic aspects of the disease. They had not learned to recognize the presence and sources of nonspecific musculoskeletal tension and fatigue within themselves or how to alleviate this tension and fatigue. Because of this, they were unsuccessful in altering the underlying disease process itself. Self-management programs need to move beyond reducing illness behaviors to regulating the psychobiological processes contributing to bodily well-being. This is not necessarily a straightforward task, as illustrated by the following case:

> Arlie is a 52-year-old with severe rheumatoid arthritis who was admitted to an inpatient psychiatry program for treatment of depression. At admission she exhibited the symptoms diagnostic of major depressive disorder (loss of interest in living, loss of weight, insomnia, and anhedonia or the inability to experience pleasure). Her arthritic symptoms were severe and required methotrexate, a powerful immunosuppressant, to control the pain, swelling and stiffness. Methotrexate is a toxic drug and its prolonged use can lead to lung disease, bone marrow suppression, liver disease, and death. In Arlie's case, the prolonged use of methotrexate had led to some dangerous changes in her liver function and she was advised to "find other ways" to control her arthritic symptoms. While on the unit, her depression was treated with paroxetine (Paxil).
>
> Arlie was severely troubled by ongoing marital difficulties which made her understanding of maintaining an internal sense of bodily well-being difficult. Her present husband was an oil industry executive and had a very strong and domineering personality. His life was his work and he seldom spent time at home. He kept business life and finances to himself. Arlie found it difficult to stand up to her husband and his success; this coupled with her arthritic deformities made her feel unwanted and unloved. She had tried fluoxetine (Prozac) for 2 years but decided to take herself off it because of the negative press the drug was receiving. She had also visited a marital counselor with her husband but nothing came of it. Her husband felt that the present episode of depression was being triggered by the methotrexate and he could not accept having a role to play in the illness.

Arlie's severe disease condition and marital situation made treatment through somatic awareness a formidable task. Some individuals are able to develop and maintain an inner somatic awareness while simultaneously facing stressful interpersonal demands and some individuals are not able to do so. Some patients have to get better control of their lives before a significant degree of somatic awareness becomes attainable. Usually patients exhibit the "two steps forward, one step backward" scenario as they simultaneously struggle with acquiring a new sense of bodily well-being while making adjustments in the thinking and behavioral styles that are contributing to their symptom condition. This patient needed to be especially diligent in monitoring herself in the presence of her husband and children:

> While on the inpatient unit, Arlie was introduced to somatic awareness as a means of gaining control of her arthritic pain and swelling. She was encouraged to utilize relaxation, reading, and aquacize [an in-pool exercise program] as a means of gaining an inner understanding of bodily ease. She was initially very enthusiastic with the concept as it seemed to provide her with a sense of self-control over her body, even though it did little to resolve feelings of anger and resentment toward her husband. Arlie insisted that she was satisfied with the therapeutic strategy, as she believed there was little or no hope that we could successfully change her husband's attitudes and behavior. For the first few weeks of treatment, her stated use of somatic awareness seemed to be producing miraculous effects. Following consultation with her rheumatologist, she was able to slowly discontinue the methotrexate, her liver functions returned to normal, and the pain and swelling disappeared. She expressed both surprise and joy with the lessening of pain, and she felt that the problem was "beat." Even her husband was pleased with the changes and was trying to be a more attentive and supportive spouse. She joined an aquatic class as well as a community volunteer group and was almost doing too much to keep the disease process in check.

The initial positive results with this patient were short-lived and she exhibited a return of the arthritic symptoms. One event in particular precipitated the relapse:

> After several weeks of feeling that her arthritis was in remission and "under control," Arlie began to feel that her life had returned to a "predisease" state. Intellectually, she seemed to have the situation well in hand. Unfortunately, emotionally she did not. Her husband and family drifted into their earlier patterns of behavior and began to treat her as they did prior to the worsening of her arthritis. She was expected to function in the social aspects of her husband's business life as well as assume the family expectations of a "normal grandmother." During one social activity, she suddenly became disoriented and dizzy, and momentarily lost her vision. Although worried about the possibility of a stroke, she managed to hide her symptoms until she returned home. Her family physician advised her on the phone to take herself to emergency at the local

hospital. She finally made it to the hospital but a thorough medical examination revealed no evidence of stroke or heart failure. She remained ill for several days.

Over the next few weeks, she became depressed and experienced a return of the arthritic pain and swelling. She cried frequently and felt that she could not go on any more. She was discouraged with the somatic awareness approach and returned to using methotrexate, vowing that she had to rely on medication as she could not rely on her family. She was once again angry at needing medications, angry about her arthritis, and angry about being a "family doormat."

This case illustrates a number of challenges patients face in using somatic awareness in the management of symptoms associated with chronic disease conditions. Individuals manage their illness on the basis of their subjective understanding of symptoms. This patient had always operated within a purely biomedical model of arthritis, viewing her arthritis as an incurable condition for which nothing could be done, other than taking medication to alleviate pain. She experienced her physical symptoms impassively and her body operated, in her view, independent from her thoughts, feelings, and level of bodily tension. Although she experienced an initial period of success, the sudden return of her symptoms was extremely disappointing and led her to believe that there was nothing more she could do. Expanding a patient's understanding of arthritis to include the experiential aspects of muscle *tension* constitutes a significant conceptual shift in inner reality and takes more than one experience with symptom improvement.

The outcome with this patient, as with all individuals with chronic disease, is both ongoing and encouraging. Today she has a better grasp of the multiple determinants of her disease, recognizes the importance of relaxation and moderate exercise, and is developing a more accepting attitude toward herself and her family. Her husband, in her words, "is trying to change." Arlie's continued progress will depend on her ability to maintain an inner bodily awareness and to self-soothe her body, especially the arthritic regions, as often as she can—until the awareness becomes virtually an automatic aspect of her being. Prior to therapy she organized all her self-perceptions around the need to maintain self-control. She understood bodily control to be best achieved by ignoring the body at all costs. Allowing bodily information into consciousness was experienced as a sign of personal weakness rather than strength. In her words, "If I learned to relax, my world would fall apart."

There was another very significant dynamic issue operating in

Arlie's mind that is seen in patients who are struggling to understand their role in managing chronic disease. For the first time in her life, Arlie was being encouraged to take control of her body. Having her understand arthritis and her body in this fashion meant to her that she was somehow responsible for the disease itself. She was already experiencing self-doubt, guilt, depression, and loneliness in the context of marital and mother–daughter issues. Requiring her to take full psychobiological responsibility for the arthritis in the context of an inattentive family represented an added burden that she did not need.

We have to come to terms with the personal responsibility issue. It is not Arlie's *fault* that she has a genetic vulnerability for arthritis or that she has the illness. It is also not her husband's fault that she is having difficulty managing the condition. Conversely, it is a mistake to conclude that because of genetics or marital issues, there is nothing she can do to manage the illness. Systemic biopsychosocial models view causality in a circular and dynamic fashion, thus making it meaningless to try and pinpoint the cause of this patient's condition to a specific genetic or psychosocial factor. We can't as yet influence the system through genetics. However, much can be done by having the arthritic patient recognize the potential healing influence of bodily self-soothing. Family members also need to accept that they are part of the solution and that there is much they can do to create a healing atmosphere for their loved one.

FATIGUE IN MULTIPLE SCLEROSIS

Chronic fatigue is an extremely common but neglected subjective symptom reported across all forms of immune system illnesses. Arthritic patients complain of persistent fatigue, fibromyalgia patients are characterized by nonrestorative sleep, and chronic fatigue syndrome patients have fatigue as the defining symptom. In this section, I will examine the symptom of fatigue as experienced by patients with multiple sclerosis (MS). Fatigue may be the single most troubling and disabling symptom experienced by MS sufferers. It can be described by some patients as overwhelming in nature and different from the fatigue that occurred when the patient was healthy. Other MS patients, however, may only mention fatigue when asked to do so. Chronic fatigue is characterized by poor tolerance of any kind of exertion, is often present upon awakening, and can be relieved by a 5- to 10-minute nap. Fatigue can be brought on by having a hot bath—an observation that led to the development of the "hot bath test." The test was once used diagnostically for individuals who were suspected of having MS but who failed to show neurological signs on examination. It was assumed that the hot bath activated MS-associated symptoms. The test has since been abandoned because of its unreliability and the fact that it sometimes resulted in permanent neurological deficits in MS patients.

MS is a neurological disease of the CNS. MS, like rheumatoid arthritis, is generally not seen as having a significant psychobiological involvement. There are clinical indications, however, that MS patients routinely use bodily signs and symptoms to their advantage to monitor their health. Although a variety of symptoms are used in this capacity, the symptom of fatigue is especially suited for determining psychological well-being, functional capacity, physical strength, and overall level of health.

MS is a disease with a fluctuating or progressive clinical course and is associated with multiple lesions in the white matter of the CNS. MS typically occurs in adults aged 15 to 55 years of age. The disease damages the myelin, the insulating cover of the CNS, and is characterized by demyelinating plaques. The onset of a symptom is linked to the breakdown of the myelin covering the neuron followed by the formation of a plaque or scarring in the area where the myelin has been destroyed. It is believed that as a consequence of disease progression, the scarring accumulates and limits recovery. The plaques occur throughout the white matter of the CNS and are especially common in the periventricular white matter.

The cause of MS is a mystery. The suspicion is that it might involve both viruses and an autoimmune reaction. The affected person's immune system, for some unknown reason, initiates an attack against its own myelin or insulating sheath. The earliest detectable bodily event is a breakdown of the blood–brain barrier in association with inflammation, which itself is believed to be immune mediated. Both the demyelination and the inflammation are hypothesized to contribute to symptom development (McDonald, Miller, & Thompson, 1994). After a period of approximately 1 month, the blood–brain barrier leakage ceases and the edema is restored. Scarring and axon loss are the residual effects of the active disease episode.

The clinical outcome of MS is rarely fatal; the majority of patients experience an illness course characterized by on-again, off-again symptom patterns. What is most characteristic about MS is the variability of its symptomatology and clinical course (Poser, 1994). Symptoms are numerous and variable; they include fatigue, bladder and bowel difficulties, backache, motor weakness, paresthesias, visual impairment, nystagmus, dysarthria, tremor, ataxia, dizziness, sexual dysfunction, pain, depression and anxiety, insomnia, spasticity, paraparesis, and cognitive dysfunction. There is no unique profile of cognitive deficits associated with MS that distinguishes it from other neurological disorders. Magnetic resonance imaging (MRI) is the preferred test of choice because it is more sensitive to detecting plaques in the CNS. However, demyelination as pictured on the MRI exhibits only modest correlations with neuropsychological impairment.

MS is highly variable and unpredictable across individuals. A course may run from occasional symptomatological exacerbations to a constant and progressively worsening form. The illness tends to follow one of four patterns. Approximately 20% of individuals will manifest a benign form, with few exacerbations and complete or nearly complete remissions. Another 25% of individuals exhibit a relapsing–remitting form that is similar to the benign form except that the exacerbations of symptoms are more severe. Some 40% of MS individuals experience a more severe relapsing–progressive form, characterized by well-defined attacks and worsening across attacks. The remaining 15% of MS sufferers experience a slowly progressive disease condition without remissions. There appears to be definite differences in coping attitudes between MS patients in the chronic progressive state and those in the remitting state. MS patients in the chronic progressive state exhibit more frustration with daily activities, coping with symptoms, and ability to work than patients in remission (Evers & Karnilowicz, 1996).

There is no single specific diagnostic test for MS. Making a firm diagnosis can be extremely difficult, especially when the symptoms do not conform to anatomical boundaries or physiological data. Often symptoms may last only a minute or two and subjective symptoms may not be confirmed by objective signs. The MRI is the preferred method for imaging the brain to detect the presence of scarring associated with MS. However, the relationship between identified plaques and disease severity is far from perfect. MS can never be diagnosed solely on the basis of an MRI because some patients with MRI-identified lesions do not have MS and a small percentage of patients who do have MS do not show MRI lesions. There is sometimes evidence of the disease process in the absence of clinical manifestation. Lesions seen at autopsy often greatly outnumber those that have been localized on the basis of the patients' signs and symptoms of neurological dysfunction. Even more puzzling is the fact that autopsies have revealed lesions in asymptomatic patients that based on their location would presumably have been especially likely to give rise to abnormal signs. Apparently the recurrence of old symptoms is more common than the appearance of new ones. It is possible that the lesions can be activated or remain dormant depending upon the presence or absence of precipitating factors.

There is no cure for MS, nor is there any generally accepted, truly efficacious specific treatment for MS. For believers in the autoimmune theory, immunomodulatory therapy has been used extensively and includes such agents as azathioprine, cyclophoasphamide, and cyclosporine. However, there is no convincing evidence that any of these agents significantly retards or arrests the progression of the disease. A large-scale study (Hall, Compston, & Scolding, 1997) involved the injection of interferon-B under double-blind controlled conditions. Interferon beta-1a was injected intramuscularly once a week for 2 years into individuals with relapsing–remitting or relapsing–progressive MS. Individuals in the study had disability scores of 1 (minimal symptoms, no disability) to 3.5 (minimal to moderate disability, fully ambulatory). There was a statistically significant reduction in the number and severity of relapses, although it was not associated with any reduction in disability. The only generally accepted treatment for exacerbation is the use of adrenocorticosteroids but long-term use is not recommended.

A link between psychological stress, fatigue, and MS onset is more than possible. There is a suspicion that stress-related fatigue precipitates changes in the immune system that are associated with both onset and relapse. Admittedly, it is equally plausible that stress and fatigue are the result rather than the cause of disease activity. Warren, Warren, and Cockerill (1991) compared relapsing and remitting patients in terms of their perceived fatigue 3 months prior to interview. Suitable subjects had to be either (1) in the midst of an exacerbation or (2) in remission for at least 6 months. Those in exacerbation reported more fatigue (63.2%) than those in remission (43.2%). Incidence of fatigue was quite high for both groups, making it impossible to determine which comes first, fatigue or relapse. At this point in our understanding of MS, it is best to view stress and fatigue systemically, that is, as subsystems that contribute to bodily dysregulation and that need to be regulated in order to restore bodily harmony and health.

Fatigue is a very common symptom outside of MS. A British survey reported that 38% of respondents attending general practice in Britain had scores above the cutoff for "substantial fatigue" (Pawlikowska et al., 1994). Close to 60% of the sample attributed their fatigue to psychological (e.g., anxiety, depression) and psychosocial causes (e.g., work, family, lifestyle) Prolonged or severe fatigue was often accompanied by reports of muscle pain. Fatigue is found across the autoimmune disorders. For example, fatigue is almost universal with fibromyalgia sufferers, and especially pronounced during disease activity. In rheumatoid arthritis, for another example, fatigue is said to peak 4.5 hours after arising, to improve with disease treatment, and to be absent in remission (Wolfe, Hawley, & Wilson, 1996). The fatigue is generally viewed as resulting from the disease process and accompanying symptoms (e.g., sleep disturbance, pain, depression) rather than causing the disease processes.

It is unknown whether the fatigue associated with MS has similar origins to the fatigue observed in chronic fatigue syndrome (CFS). This is an extremely important issue. If the fatigue has a similar origin, then it will be easier to help MS sufferers to shift their attributions of the causes of the fatigue from purely disease factors to psychobiological factors. It is known that patients with CFS who harbor strong disease attributions for the fatigue have a poor prognosis of recovery (Joyce, Hotopf, & Wessely, 1997). The same may be true for MS sufferers. In a comparison of fatigue in MS patients and CFS patients, the severity of reported fatigue levels was similar for the two groups (Vercoulen et al., 1996). Fatigue was present in 85% of the MS patients and 100% of the CFS patients at least once a week. For both groups, however, it is not known whether the experienced fatigue is similar or dissimilar to the fatigue associated with normal tiredness that affects muscles after exercise or other physical exertion. MS fatigue may come on faster than ordinary fatigue.

That fatigue in MS is psychobiologically determined is only a hypothesis. The biomedical view holds that the fatigue associated with MS is caused by neurological factors different from the causes of ordinary fatigue. The biomedical view holds that MS fatigue is determined centrally—that is, it develops from weakened impulses associated with demyelinated nerves. In this view, MS fatigue reflects a form of physiological, rather than psychobiological, exhaustion. The nerves momentarily lose their ability to conduct impulses in a normal fashion. Thus fatigue of motor nerves is seen as responsible for symptoms of general weakness, painful muscle spasms, incoordination, and shakiness, while fatigue of sensory nerves may contribute to blurred vision, numbness, and other sensory symptoms. However, the physiological-exhaustion hypothesis is also speculative. A study by Fisk, Pontefract, Rivto, Archibald, and Murray (1994) found no relationship between severity of reported fatigue and ratings of neurological impairment, suggesting that the determinants of fatigue are not necessarily the outcome of neurological parameters.

Fatigue in MS affects more than the patient's symptoms. It interferes with the individual's ability to function in all aspects of life. The Fatigue Impact Scale (Fisk et al., 1994) views fatigue as having impact on cognitive function ("I feel that I cannot think clearly," "I find that I am more forgetful"), physical function ("My muscles feel much weaker than they should," "I have to limit my physical activities"), and social function ("I am more irritable and easily angered," "I engage in less sexual activity"). Thus, feelings of fatigue can quickly lead to avoidance of activity because patients view activity as causing their fatigue. Inactivity can lead to further physical deconditioning as well as to feelings of helplessness and depression. Thus chronic fatigue can interfere with all aspects of living.

Evidence that the fatigue experienced by MS sufferers may result from excess life stress is mixed. Rabins et al. (1986) asked MS patients to fill in monthly life events' diaries over a 1-year period. Of the 87 patients who participated, 23 experienced exacerbations. To determine whether increased stressful events commonly preceded an exacerbation, the researchers compared relapsing patients' scores in the month during which they reported an exacerbation to their mean scores for all previous months. Robins et al. found no significant difference. But other researchers (Grant et al., 1989) have found a significant excess of marked life stress in the 6 months previous to exacerbation onset in MS patients.

The management of fatigue is recognized as central to coping with MS. Patients are encouraged to be aware of their limits and to listen to their bodies for signs that they may need to disengage from activity and/or rest. Fatigue is often the first sign that other symptoms are about to recur. Excessive fatigue is often responsible for other symptoms such as weakness of the limbs and depression. As a typical MS patient noted, "When I get too far beyond my limits, I get over-tired, and when that happens I get depressed. I try to avoid fatigue because I feel overwhelmed and out of control" (McLaughlin & Zeeberg, 1993, p. 321).

Curiously, there are individuals with remitting MS who suffer from regular fatigue and yet can respond to extreme physical demands such as running a marathon, as the following case illustrates:

> Marci is a 37-year-old woman who first experienced MS symptoms at the age of 16 when she suffered temporary loss of vision in one eye. She was diagnosed with MS at the age of 21. At that time she was experiencing major life stress: she was holding three part-time jobs in order to pay her way through school as a medical technician. With the unexpected diagnosis of MS she was also given a grim prognosis: being wheelchair-bound within 5 years. Marci was determined not to let this happen. She decided to fight the disease by strengthening her body through diet, exercise, and marathon running. Fitness became her primary way of coping with the disease. Some 16 years later she completed the grueling Boston Marathon and shows no progression of the disease.
>
> Marci is presently married with no children. She was advised

to avoid the additional stress and fatigue that having children would bring about. Her fatigue and other symptoms are mild at the moment. "Each day I have a lot of spasms in my leg. . . . Actually the spasms may not really be in my leg . . . it may be my brain indicating that something is wrong in the leg when in fact there is not. . . . My leg feels like a rubber band is tied around it and is being pulled in all directions. It can happen in one leg or the other, although it is usually at the end of the day that it is at its worst such as when I am driving home from work. I use Tegretol [carbamazepine–an anticonvulsant medication used for neurological symptoms] and a hot bath to lessen the symptoms. Tegretol works well and surprisingly so does a hot bath. I know a hot bath is supposed to make the symptoms worse, but in my case the spasm sensations disappear . . . it is the cold I hate."

When asked if personality/coping might contribute to her symptoms, Marci replied negatively. She believes that MS is caused by a virus. However, she admitted to having a "triple Type A" personality, which in her case reflects a general inability to relax, self-initiated pressure, and extreme competitiveness. She stated that she was brought up to believe one should always work hard. She believes that her Type A personality, rather than contributing to the MS, provides her with the inner strength to fight the disease. She has a brother who is much more debilitated with MS, and she believes that in large part his debilitation reflects a lack of fighting spirit. She openly admitted to not knowing how to relax, other than through strenuous exercise. She also has a working hypothesis that the demanding exercise associated with marathon training suppresses her immune system and thereby reduces the presence of MS activity.

Her personal beliefs are very close to those individuals described earlier who suffered from CFS. Her self-admitted Type A personality reflected a strong desire for accomplishment and equally strong standards for personal performance. During her early years, while maintaining three jobs, she was leading an overextended and overcommitted lifestyle and feeling pressed for time. Although she now listens to her body and rests when tired, there are times when she will push through the fatigue no matter how tired she feels. In earlier days she can recall times when working out in a fitness center that she would have to hang on to the equipment because she was too tired to stand alone. During the running of a marathon, she uses a string tied around the front of her shoe to lift her toes to prevent foot dragging and stumbling from fatigue.

Marci's way of coping is interesting in terms of my discussion of somatic awareness. She appears to integrate aspects of the concept into her coping with MS in recognizing fatigue levels and she also exhibits aspects of avoiding bodily information, especially when she feels that it is necessary to get on with living. Maybe she has found the right balance of awareness and nonawareness. Her fighting spirit, in her words, is what gets her out of bed in the morning and on with the day, regardless of how her body feels. At the same time, she does listen to her body. When her fatigue levels are especially high she makes certain to get extra sleep. When running, she pays attention to her breathing and uses imagery to increase blood flow to regions that are hurting. She uses hot water to relax her legs and also regularly visits a masseuse.

This individual also began using relaxation as a means of lessening her leg spasms. Her use of muscle relaxation to control peripheral spasms is relevant to the earlier discussion of whether symptoms in MS are central or peripheral in origin. In this instance, the issue is whether the perceived spasm involves psychobiological determinants such as tension in leg muscle or is the result of CNS changes leading to irregularity in the outflow of the motor nerves. After a few practice sessions she was able to prevent through relaxation the spasm sensations if they were mild. Although her control does not prove that peripheral muscle relaxation is involved, her newfound ability is consistent with the use of somatic awareness to achieve this control. She still had difficulty using somatic awareness if the spasms became severe; she generally copes with severe spasm by ignoring the sensation for as long as possible, a strategy that she admits is not necessarily effective.

Somatic awareness needs to be systematically explored across the different variants of MS. Individuals with the relapsing–remitting variant of the condition might have greater opportunity than individuals with progressive MS for recognizing subtle changes within their environment and within themselves that mark the transition from one stage to the other. The pursuance of somatic awareness in patients with chronic progressive MS is equally important. Like any individual with chronic disease, he/she is required to fend for him/herself during many periods of worsening symptoms. Given that the disease is progressive, there is a very real concern that the appearance and/or worsening of any symptom signifies disease progression and further loss of independence. Any action these individuals can take to maintain their present level of bodily empowerment is critical for reducing the uncertainty of the future.

THE EXISTENTIAL SHIFT IN CANCER

The discussion of arthritis and multiple sclerosis suggests that bodily awareness and self-soothing work best when individuals can "let go" at multiple levels within themselves. Thus they learn not only to relax physically but they also learn to relax or let go of other emotionally and physically destructive aspects of themselves. The same situation characterizes cancer patients who have been observed to enter a period of disease reversal or spontaneous remission. Spontaneous disappearance of cancer has been documented in hundreds of cases. The initial description of cancer disappearance in the absence of treatment as *spontaneous* implied that the recoveries occurred without reason or cause (Challis & Stam, 1990). Consequently, there was little interest in identifying factors responsible for such occurrences. However, this attitude has changed dramatically. Rather than viewing these occurrences as mysterious or inexplicable, clinicians are beginning to better understand and harness the processes in use by these individuals.

Spontaneous remission of a number of diseases may be more commonplace than is generally assumed. Pincus (1996) hypothesized that spontaneous remission may actually be the normal outcome for most diseases:

> In at least one disease, rheumatoid arthritis . . . , considerable evidence indicates that most people who meet criteria for having rheumatoid arthritis probably experience spontaneous remission and do not develop the disease. . . . This evidence is derived from population studies, that is, studies conducted in the community in which all individuals in a defined population are examined. In two such studies conducted in the 1960s, . . . 1 to 2 percent of the population were identified as having swollen joints, meeting the criteria for rheumatoid arthritis. However, when these individuals were reviewed 3 to 5 years later, fewer than 50 percent of them still met the criteria, and most had no disease at all. In short, in more than 50 percent of the people who showed the clinical signs of rheumatoid arthritis, the symptoms had disappeared—had gone into remission. (p. 66)

Observations regarding individuals with rheumatoid arthritis may hold for life-threatening diseases such as cancer. It has been suggested, for example, that the formation of cancer cells is a common everyday occurrence in humans and that most of them do not develop into cancer because of the immune system's "surveillance" properties. Spontaneous remission is known to occur with cancer. O'Regan and Hirshberg (1993) summarized the literature dealing with 1,386 cases of spontaneous remission of various forms of cancer. They provide a wide discussion of possible explanations for the remissions, including fevers, infections, spirituality, meditation, diet, herbs, and other factors. Individuals who have experienced spontaneous remission generally report a qualitative shift in the way they perceive themselves and their bodies, and in the way they live life. Generally, they report abandoning an extremely self-sacrificing lifestyle in favor of a self-soothing lifestyle in which they take care of themselves rather than others. Their adjustments generally include a change in core belief and value systems.

The experts all seem to agree that one's chance of survival improves to the extent that one can find a new way of perceiving oneself in the context of living with the disease. Such profound changes, it is thought, are most likely to facilitate shifts toward positive emotionality and resultant immunoenhancement (Dafter, 1996).

> When people experience a major medical illness, a person's usual patterns of self-experience are shattered through the activation of powerful and disorienting emotions. *The fear and other powerful emotions evoked when one confronts annihilation from death may initiate in many people an unsolicited life review and force them to emotionally evaluate the unfinished elements of their living.* (p. 68)

From such emotions people would gain essential information about what areas in their present lives need to be improved in quality, and gain as well a powerful motivation to make inner and outer life changes to redirect their lives in new directions. The content of a person's review might emphasize either the psychological past or the present, depending on the person's unique biopsychosocial history, place in the human life cycle, and personality organization.

Michael Lerner (1994) of the Commonweal Cancer Help Program suggests that the significant common denominator in cases of spontaneous remission is the extent to which individuals are able to make a complete break with their previous ways of thinking, behaving, and living. Individuals who experience spontaneous remission seem to have also undergone an existential transformation or shift in their approach to life. This hypothesis originated from the observations of Ikemi and colleagues (Ikemi, Nakagawa, Nakagawa, & Sugita, 1975) of five cases of spontaneous remission in Japan. Two of these cases are presented to illustrate the existential changes which these individuals underwent following their cancer diagnosis:

> A 64-year-old man with a histologically confirmed cancer of the upper right jaw refused all medical treatment. A Shinto preacher,

he felt that "this is God's will and I will have no complaint about it. Whatever should happen will just happen." Ikemi and colleagues (1975) report:

> Ten days after the "sentence of cancer," he visited the president of the religious organization who said to him: "Remember that you are an invaluable asset for our church." This made him feel very happy and he shed tears of joy all the way back home. Since this moving experience, his hoarseness [a symptom of the cancer] began to improve. . . . Today Dr. F. says: "The cancer of this patient seems to be practically cured. When I looked into the vocal cord through the larnygoscope, the tumor was gone." (pp. 184–185)

A 63-year-old farm wife was diagnosed at 58 with histologically confirmed extensive metastatic adenocarcinoma of the stomach. Palliative surgery was performed and she was given 1 to 3 months to live. The patient had worked extremely hard all her life on the farm. Reports Ikemi (Ikemi et al., 1975), "A drastic change took place in her pattern of life since she became ill. Before surgery she led a life of sacrifice for the family as mentioned above, while after surgery the attitude of the whole family has been very considerate and kind toward her. She was set free from many years of a self-sacrificing way of life, and was now protected by the love of the family" (p. 186).

Both these individuals let go to some extent of a previous lifestyle in favor of one characterized by acceptance, love from others, and love for others.

Lerner (1994) reviewed a second study (van Baalen, de Vries, & Gondrie, 1987) of spontaneous remission of seven patients that reached the conclusion that in all cases a "more or less radical existential shift" had taken place. A communality of this group is that they recognized the importance of taking care of themselves rather than others. Feelings of dependency and helplessness shifted toward increased autonomy and hopefulness:

> The most significant correlates of SRC [spontaneous recovery, in advanced cancer] seem to be behavioral and sensory changes and shifts along the depression and autonomy axes. However, also belief and trust in medical procedures, among them alternative medicine, shifts in mental constructs about cancer and its treatment, existential shifts and improvement of social support and the quality of interpersonal relationships are significant. . . .
>
> The generally high scores of SRC patients [on depression] seem to suggest that allowing oneself to experience depression temporarily, rather

than repressing such a state or staying in a depression, is associated with SRC. . . .

Existential shifts may not be in a direction commonly regarded as "positive," such as an increased experience of meaning in life and so-called spiritual or religious conversions. This is demonstrated by two of our patients. Their existential shifts could easily be misinterpreted as "negative" in the sense of aggressiveness and being obnoxious. (p. 188)

Berland (1995) explored through qualitative research the reasons cancer patients provided for surviving the disease. He interviewed 33 individuals who had lived for an extended time despite having received a "terminal" medical prognosis (defined by their physicians/ oncologists as having 20% or less probability of surviving 5 years or longer). At the time of the study, 28 of the 33 participants had lived longer than 5 years since diagnosis. None of their physicians had expected these patients to be alive at the time of the interview for the study.

As a first step in assessing subject attributions as to why they thought they were still alive, Berland had subjects complete a "medi-cine pie chart." The chart is a tool for measuring the specific factors to which respondents attribute recovery. A composite pie chart revealed that the five dominant attributions in rank order were: support of fam-ily and friends, attitudinal change, medical treatment, spirituality, and alternative treatments. The essential source of healing as seen by 28 out of 33 subjects involved the examination of core values and the most meaningful aspects of their lives. Berland provided examples of numerous cases in which people experienced despair, depression, ter-ror, and suicidal feelings in reaction to their illness. The soul-searching process of working with these feelings resulted in dramatic attitudinal, spiritual, and existential shifts, with associated changes in core emo-tional self-experience. These inner shifts were also associated with the outer expression of new values, which were made manifest through the patients' relationships with loved ones and with God, as well as in the creation of new lifestyles.

Berland reports that more than half the participants in the study attributed their healing to an existential shift in their perspectives about life. The changes involved more than attitudinal factors and were truly existential or spiritual in nature. Their perceptions about their lives clearly took on a new texture, and all of them reported a sense of feeling fulfilled and of being part of something larger than themselves. They claimed to have been forever and deeply changed by the transfor-mation that occurred. They felt that their lives and well-being depended on remaining true to their new understandings about themselves and their priorities. They began to live a life committed to the expression of what they considered their true natures and their own needs. The following patient statement illustrates this outlook:

"True full healing, if you want to heal the being, you need to face yourself utterly, honestly, and fully, and to be there in every way you need and to listen to your truth, which is all the same thing I'm saying, and to honor it no matter what. Anything less than that, you're going to get what you pay for. . . . It's the commitment 100 percent to never not live your truth, to never find an excuse, and I think that is the real key . . . to live, to live fully." (p. 12)

The individuals in the Berland study of spontaneous remission all found individualized ways to take better care of themselves—physically, psychologically, and spiritually. Their heightened awareness clearly had more to do with the psychological self than the physical self. However, I feel that somatic awareness, although not discussed by Berland and his subjects, is a significant component of the solace and inner calm that many of these individuals achieved:

"I thought I would probably kill myself. I became extremely depressed. It's real hard to say what happened, but what did happen was one day I woke up and wasn't interested in being sick anymore. I became interested in making willow furniture. . . . I became another person. I wasn't the person who worked really hard and did all this. I became a much more contemplative person, I became a much more creative person, a much more quiet person, and I started really small, really small." (p. 14)

One additional example illustrates the spiritual/mystical associations that accompanied the bodily calm in some of these patients:

"And this light came down over me, and it was very, very, very bright as it went across my eyes. . . . It lasted for 15 or 20 seconds . . . and I was incredibly peaceful. I was just as calm as I've ever been in my life. Two minutes before that, I'd been as terrified as I'd ever been in my life. . . . Being rather mystical and spiritual, I kind of hung onto those things. . . . It meant that my prayers were being answered, maybe not in the way in which I had asked for them to be, but in a very comforting way. . . . It gave me a universal connection." (Berland, 1995, p. 14)

We should not forget that spontaneous remission is still a relatively rare event. Those individuals fortunate enough to recover have had to experienced some very fundamental change in their psychoneuroimmunology. We still need to identify the construct that links the existential and immunological realities of the patient. We need to know, for example, whether a combination of letting go of psychological issues, decreasing bodily tension, and employing intentional and directed self-soothing is capable of taking inner healing to a higher level.

A personal story of recovery from cancer is found in *Mind, Fantasy, and Healing: One Woman's Journey from Conflict and Illness to Wholeness and Health,* by Alice Epstein (1989). She developed a form of a kidney cancer called hypernephroma. Her left kidney had a large tumor and the cancer had spread to her lungs. In describing the origins of this condition, Alice believed that she fit almost perfectly the Type C character pattern that I discussed earlier. Alice characterized herself as feeling helpless and hopeless in the face of stress, of not expressing her feelings, of being extremely sympathetic and helpful toward others, and of finding it hard to express anger. She was also extremely critical of herself and prone to belittling her accomplishments, including obtaining a doctoral degree. She interpreted her unwillingness to express anger as a deeply rooted fear of disapproval and rejection.

> I, like others with a cancer-prone personality, learned early on that it was very important to please my mother, and this model of relationship carried over into my way of relating to the world. Pleasing others therefore became the *major motivation* in my life. My orientation toward others resulted in empathy and sensitivity to the needs of others, but it brought me pain because it was too extreme and unmodulated. As a result I could not separate myself from the sorrows of others. I suffered especially when anything bad happened to my sister or my daughters. I also felt unhappy because I was constantly attending to the needs of others while no one was attending to my needs. (p. 25)

Alice approached her personal healing with a passion that others might also find difficult to sustain. She allowed nothing to interrupt her self-healing. She would meditate several times during the day: early in the morning, before breakfast, at noon, at sunset, and before going to bed. Her meditation began with a few minutes of quiet in which she tensed and relaxed each part of her body. This was followed by Vipassana meditation which involves attending to the breath. Next she added a form of visualization, by watching her breath. The process took at least 45 minutes and often longer, which means she was meditating close to 4 hours per day.

This intense body meditation was just the beginning of Alice's transformation. She developed a level of spirituality and intellectual connectedness characterized by letting go at all levels of her existential being. She took the position that despite her love for her husband, she would leave him if she felt that was necessary to improve her life.

In other words, if my life were on the line in a decision between relating and living, I would choose to live. It was a very important insight, because in the past I had always made the opposite decision. The knowledge that it would be different now was a source of great strength to me. . . . I believe that this assurance to myself that at last I could let my life come first was the beginning of the motivation that I needed to live. Finally, I wanted to live just for me. (p. 65)

Other changes she made included coming to terms with mother–daughter love–hate feelings, her relationship with her father, self-destructive forces within herself, the content of dreams, and working through a number of negative self-personalities. All of the changes she made to her physical and psychological self resulted in a complete remission of her disease. Alice was fortunate to have a full range of healing resources within her reach. She lived in an intellectual community and had ready access to wide expertise dealing with visualization, meditation, spirituality, existentialism, and relaxation. She also was supported in these endeavors by her husband, himself a psychologist with a thorough understanding of mind–body issues.

Other cancer specialists believe in the need for significant psychological change for maximizing recovery from cancer. Lawrence LeShan (Bolletino & LeShan, 1995) developed a form of intensive "marathon" psychotherapy for use with cancer patients. The therapy takes place over 6 consecutive days and is designed to bring about rapid changes in lifestyle and personality. LeShan believes that the patient needs to make a significant existential shift toward determining what makes him or her feel alive and then find activities that promote these life-serving feelings. LeShan believes that for any plan to be effective, it must address the whole person. That is, it must involve the person's unique physical, psychological, and spiritual needs—the person's best ways of being, relating, and creating. Inner changes and changes in lifestyle must be made together to reinforce each other.

The majority of people faced with cancer may not be comfortable with psychotherapeutic approaches that require a complete overhaul of their psychological being. They may like life as it is—minus the life-threatening disease. Learning to make psychobiological adjustments within present lifestyle circumstances should be as effective in promoting healing as major lifestyle change *as long as* the individual is able to achieve significant levels of bodily well-being. Somatic awareness might serve as a guide as to what kinds of changes or adjustments need to be made in one's relationship with oneself and with others. Somatic awareness can serve as an experiential frame of reference for integrating information from our more rational mind in dealing with disease.

For example, it can focus cancer patients on the importance of taking care of themselves as opposed to others, of moderating the adverse effects of personality attributes, and of enhancing social support systems—all of which can enhance feelings of psychobiological well-being.

Somatic awareness is offered as an integrative rather than a curative concept in dealing with cancer and other diseases. Each individual must find his/her own path in dealing with such a disease and no one can really know how he/she will react until faced with such an experience. Lerner (1994), in responding to the hypothetical question "What would I do if it were me?", offered a number of relevant thoughts. First and foremost he said: "I would be paying a great deal of attention to the *inner healing process* that I hope that the diagnosis would trigger in me. I would be giving careful thought to what had meaning for me now—just what in my life I wanted to let go of and what I wanted to keep" (p. 532). He noted, at a practical level, the careful selection of a mainstream physician and conventional treatments and the importance of working with both to augment their effectiveness. In addition, he would use a number of complementary therapies, augment a regular nutritional program, use traditional Chinese medicine, and spend more time with other people, nature, and God. In closing this carefully offered advice, he emphasized that with cancer "there is no single right choice for all of us, but there are surely right choices for each of us." In a similar spirit of hope, I offer somatic awareness as a concept to guide individuals in making experiential choices based on what is for the moment our best understanding of the processes involved.

Group Healing

In closing, I will comment on the present tendency to study the potential benefits of psychology in treating cancer through the practice of group therapy. Interest in the healing benefits of group therapy began with a report from Spiegel and colleagues (Spiegel, Bloom, Kraemer, & Gottheil, 1989). They generated initial interest in group psychotherapy with the demonstration that patients with metastatic breast cancer who were seen in "weekly supportive group therapy" had significantly longer survival than a group of matched controls who were randomly assigned to treatments that did not include the psychotherapy program. Spiegel et al. (1989, p. 890) described the supportive group psychotherapy as emphasizing "living as fully as possible, improving communication with family members and doctors, facing and mastering fears about death and dying, and controlling pain and other symptoms." The authors argue that social support mediates how individuals cope with stress, which can improve health outcome. The supportive group therapy provided a place for these patients "to belong and express their feelings. . . . [They] felt an intense bonding with one another and a sense of acceptance through sharing a common dilemma" (p. 890). The group therapy seemed to enable the cancer patients to comply more effectively with treatment, which included improving appetite and diet as well as maintaining exercise and normal routine activity, through a reduction in depression and pain.

There is some research support showing that improvements in cancer survival time following group therapy are associated with improvement in immune system function. Fawzy et al. (1990a, 1990b) provided follow-up data on 66 patients with malignant melanoma who underwent standard initial surgical treatment. One-half were randomized to a control group; the other half underwent a structured psychiatric group intervention within several months of the original diagnosis and initial surgical treatment. Groups of 7 to 10 patients met in 90-minute sessions once a week to focus on four components: (1) education about melanoma, sun protection, and healthy nutrition; (2) stress management, including personal stress awareness and relaxation techniques; (3) coping and problem-solving skills; and (4) psychological support from staff and other patients.

At 6 months, the group participants had improved coping ability, reduced psychological distress, and improved immune function. The treatment group subjects maintained greater numbers and activity of tumor-killing cells compared to the control group. The most striking results appeared 6 years after the initial diagnosis and treatment. Only 3 of the 38 patients in the psychosocial groups had died, compared with 10 of 28 in the control group. The group patients also tended to have fewer instances of recurrence; just 7 experienced recurrence compared with 13 control patients. Given the complexity of the group interventions, it is impossible to know what elements of the various therapies were most therapeutic or whether they all worked together in some fashion. Intervention may have fostered improved health habits such as more careful sun protection, better nutrition, and regular exercise. Effective coping may have improved physician–patient communication and adherence to treatment and follow-up regimens. Patients may have learned to manage stress more effectively through problem solving, changing attitudes toward minor daily stressors, or altering their physiological response to stress through relaxation techniques. All of the factors mentioned above could each have contributed in some way to reduce overall stress within these patients. The group patients also received a great deal of social support. They could express their feelings freely to an understanding and sympathetic audience and hear how others were dealing with the same disease. Somatic awareness may have been a by-product of some of these strategies (e.g., relaxation) but its use was not directly encouraged.

Those patients who used avoidance coping such as avoiding others, hiding feelings, or refusing to think about their illness tended to have more recurrence and lower survival rates. Patients who reported higher levels of emotional distress at the time of diagnosis and treatment had lower rates of recurrence and death. Patients with the highest risk were those who minimized and expressed little distress. Distress in the face of life-threatening illness is appropriate and may help motivate patients to mobilize coping resources and behaviors, but persistent denial may interfere with this essential mobilization process.

Avoidance defenses do more than reduce subjective awareness of feeling: they also reduce bodily awareness. It stands to reason that if one is unaware of subjective feelings, then one may have difficulty understanding and describing bodily feelings. If one is unaware of or does not acknowledge increased arousal due to stress or emotion, one is not able to respond appropriately and may experience prolonged periods of physiological arousal that tax the immune system and eventually result in disease.

A number of research teams are currently exploring the utility of group psychotherapy in combination with medical treatment to improve psychological adjustment and quality of life in dealing with cancer. These same research teams are exploring whether similar group interactions might strengthen the body's capacity to resist the progression of the disease. These researchers are placing their faith in the healing power of social support, arguing that therapeutic groups often have the potential to provide for greater intimate support than friends and family can offer. The question remains whether somatic awareness, when explicitly directed by the intervention process, can strengthen the individual's chances of survival. What would be the outcome, for example, of comparing social support groups that worked directly on somatic awareness training versus support groups that concentrated on the recognition and sharing of feelings? I believe that cancer patients will fare better if they are taught to practice self-soothing experiences during the course of therapy.

An advantage of the somatic awareness emphasis is that the intervention need not be practiced in groups. In fact, somatic awareness can be difficult to implement within a group format because the emphasis of discussion is generally on interpersonal rather than on intrapersonal issues. Also, many patients with cancer and other diseases are unwilling to discuss their condition in groups. These individuals need a way of understanding what they can do within their private selves to maximize inner healing resources.

Providing Hope

In closing this discussion of cancer, I want to emphasize the value of hope. The initial diagnosis of cancer is frightening and can lead to a variety of negative feelings, including confusion, fatigue, exhaustion, tension, resentfulness, and helplessness. A cancer diagnosis can result in immediate disruption of family and social lives, work, and the ability to enjoy leisure activities. It takes time to resolve the affective distress associated with a diagnosis of cancer.

Block (1997) believes that health professionals can do much to activate the inner healing resources of patients dealing with cancer. He feels that they must approach the cancer patient in a manner that brings compassion and support to the caring exchange:

> Such care, expressed in part through an unrelenting, life-affirming attitude, is neither an "extra" nor hokum. Quite the contrary. In my view, a model that is exclusively focused on cure-giving while not equally addressing caregiving is incomplete at the least. Caregiving entails an open, empathic frame of mind; it means devoting sincere, ongoing attention to and recognition of the sacredness of each individual life. I believe this heartfelt attitude, reflecting on the part of the caregiver a kind of higher self . . . is the first step in putting the person suffering from cancer or any other life-threatening illness on a path that rouses in them the energy and commitment consciously to struggle with their cancer. This is where the healing process begins. In experiencing the optimism of possibility, even in regard to life-threatening illness, people feel more whole, more alive, more engaged with life, sometimes more than ever before. People feel inspired to go on living, to fight for their life from the inside out. (p. 7)

All of a person's inner resources need to be tapped to fight the cancer illness. A sense of engagement in one's own healing can spell the difference between relapse and remission. In Block's approach, it is vital that the patient and the caregiver develop a partnership and an affinity for the treatment approach chosen. The following passage, taken from Block (1997), represents an excellent piece of wisdom for the individual with cancer who is trying to maximize inner healing resources:

> Patients also need to be encouraged to seek out all the positive support possible and eliminate negative influences in their private, public, and medical lives. This could mean getting out of friendships that lead to discontentment or exhaustion, and finding friendships that evoke feelings of mirth, tranquillity, and fulfillment. It could also mean leaving a job that feels detrimental, or a job in which one's superiors or coworkers fail to provide positive reinforcement. On certain occasions, I have written pre-

scriptions for some patients that simply read, "Fire your boss." Finally, it could also mean ending a relationship with a caregiver if that relationship is damaging and negating one's core needs and desires, both of which are necessary for a person to constructively address his or her personal/emotional and medical/biological care. (p. 23)

I must mention the need to be aware of the guilt potential associated with the various self-help treatments. Patients who are encouraged to utilize relaxation, visualization, positive thoughts, prayer, and so forth and who do not improve can be expected, unless properly prepared, to experience a deep sense of frustration and guilt that they are doing something wrong. In broad terms, the idea expressed is that if you are expected to take an active role in your treatment and you do not improve, then in some way you have failed. This is an important reason for providing patients with outlets for emotional expression related to the results of treatment.

> Coping attitudes can also be affected by the results of treatment. The basic need for self-preservation impels many people to inquire into effective cancer treatments and to consider alternatives. If the initial treatment is successful, the person is likely to emerge intact and feeling positive about the experience. If the treatment is short-lived or unsuccessful, the person is likely to feel more anxious, fearful, enraged, confused, and uncertain than before. This seems to be true no matter how well educated a person is: the cancer experience, when intensified by a metastasis, an inoperable tumor, uncontrollable pain or frequent recurrences, is an emotional roller coaster that can rattle even the most resilient human spirit. (Block, 1997, p. 14)

The psychosocial literature dealing with immune system illnesses is consistent with my central thesis of the importance of bodily self-soothing in maximizing opportunities for recovery and disease management. Although there is no solid clinical evidence that bodily awareness used in this manner will make a difference, it seems that everything we do know, both in terms of basic and applied research, points in this direction. Minimizing life events and emotion/coping styles that are associated with persistent bodily tension and fatigue are clearly indicated. Learning to let go of things and people in one's life that interfere with and/or prevent self-soothing is also critical. Bodily awareness does not necessarily have to be actively worked upon, but if it is not the person must have a clear understanding of how to activate the same psychobiological processes through other forms of conscious activity and lifestyle changes. Clinicians who attempt to work with this concept need to be especially sensitive to the patient's preferred coping styles and stage of illness. The issue should not be forced—especially when bodily sensations may portend a worsening disease condition. The need for caution, however, should not discourage the patients' bodily exploration and discovery. No harm can be caused by telling cancer patients that their disease involves some form of immunological impairment and that through somatic awareness development combined with psychotherapy and/or support groups it is possible to achieve immunoenhancement. Cancer patients have nothing to lose and everything to gain by participating actively in an integrated psychoneuroimmunological treatment program (Block, 1997). Somatic awareness remains a very fundamental experiential benchmark for determining what to let go of and what to keep in learning to cope with a diagnosis of cancer.

A final word on providing cancer patients with hope is in order. Since the literature concerning self-regulation of cancer began to appear, there have been expressions of concern that cancer victims are being provided with false hope in the form of suggestions that they can influence the course of their disease. According to these experts, it is better that they accept the reality of the disease and prepare to die. Block (1997) is outraged at this practice, stating that it amounts to bludgeoning the patient with words and gestures into a state of futility and hopelessness. It is his belief that hopelessness is often an iatrogenic or doctor-induced condition that destroys the patient's spirit, suppresses the immune system, and facilitates the patient's demise. He believes that no matter how poor the biomedical prognosis, it is better to communicate to the patient in a fashion that is likely to bolster the patient's spirit and biology. People living with cancer cannot afford to be living with a terminal disease mind-set. People need to maintain hope.

Buchholz (1997) stated that the goal of cancer treatment programs is not just a longer life but a *larger* life. Life is more than an event along a time axis—it possesses breadth and depth as well. In Buchholz's words, *"The amount of life a person has is the product of how long the person lives, how well the person lives (quantity of life), and how meaningful is the person's life"* (p. 32). Physicians who develop cancer programs must be aware of this fact and present programs that balance treatments with life values. Similarly, patients who seek a comprehensive treatment program must be aware that they need more than the perfect physician. They need to assemble a healing team who will reflect their goals of treatment. "When patient and physician can come together in this spirit, they create the possibility of *tikkun*, Hebrew for healing and transformation" (Buchholz, 1997, p. 33).

There is no magic formula for utilizing somatic awareness with cancer, other than to seek activities and treatments that facilitate an inner sense of bodily well-being and self-soothing. It is unknown how cancer works, and it remains to be empirically demonstrated that a self-regulation model based on somatic awareness might make a difference. Still, the testimonials from survivors and professionals are entirely consistent with the notion of self-soothing and immunoenhancement. Most often the reports from survivors acknowledge that changes in bodily awareness do occur as a result of newly discovered self-esteem, meaningful life activities, adjustments to diet, and networking with other patients. These testimonials integrate the best wisdom from outside oneself with the bodily wisdom within oneself.

CHAPTER 5

Helping Others Find Their Bodies

The experience of bodily well-being, although occurring in the form of private self-consciousness, is a state of being available to everyone. Somatic awareness is a form of bodily self-knowledge that a person can draw upon at any time during the waking state: at work, at rest, at play, while alone, or when in the company of others. In this closing chapter I will examine the importance of having health professionals develop somatic awareness in their patients. Such awareness can be facilitated by all health professionals, regardless of their training and treatment orientation. Health professionals from all disciplines can strengthen their healing influence by incorporating a somatic awareness perspective into their practice. Establishing somatic awareness with a patient requires collaboration between professional and patient: to be effective, today's health professional must administer treatment with the active involvement of his/her patient.

Therapists who wish to develop somatic awareness in their clinical practice must first recognize the healing potential within their patients and then encourage their patients to become equal partners in the treatment process. That is, they must do more than establish a positive professional–patient relationship: they must accept the idea that their main function as professional healers is to *empower* patients to utilize the healing forces within themselves. Without such empowerment, many patients will simply be "good patients" and do as they are told. Such an approach is not likely to generate reliable and lasting treat-

ment effects. Given that so many common chronic symptoms and illnesses are psychobiological in origin, healing interventions must be
presented within a psychobiological perspective.

This chapter begins with an examination of therapeutic touch and
biofeedback, two of the most popular alternative medicine techniques
associated with bodily sensations. Although these therapies are associated with bodily sensations and bodily self-control, they are not automatically associated with bodily well-being. This is so because of the
way in which the therapy is administered. Touch therapy is usually presented as a form of healing in which the source of healing power lies
within the therapist rather than within the patient him/herself. Similarly, biofeedback, although it seems to be about enhancing bodily self-
control, is to often administered as a high-tech intervention that the
patient "is given" in order to gain direct control of the underlying physiological system that is being used to generate the electronic feedback.
No general experience of somatic awareness is assumed to be required
for the intervention to be effective.

We will see that it is far better to present therapies involving touch
and biofeedback in the context of somatic awareness than it is to present these therapies as specific interventions that operate outside of
such awareness. The same argument would hold for the many other
bodily therapies and self-regulatory strategies, including massage,
relaxation, reflexology, hydrotherapy, and self-hypnosis. I will examine
controlled breathing in detail—mainly because I believe that a form of
effortless breathing is at the heart or "abdomen" of somatic awareness.
Although I discuss several techniques, it is important to reemphasize
my belief that all self-regulatory interventions have far greater healing
potential when presented in the larger context of enhancing personal
experiences of bodily well-being. The final segment of the chapter
offers a general invitation to health professionals to develop a somatic
awareness perspective within themselves and within their clinical practice.

HEALING ENERGY

The concept of healing energy, presented in the form of therapeutic touch, has resurfaced as one of the more popular forms of alternative medicine. In some locales touch therapy is becoming a self-
contained profession with standards, guidelines, and required accredi-
tation procedures. We have entered an era in which the caring act of
touching needs to be administered by a trained professional. This is so
because the healers believe that they are capable of achieving levels of

energy transformation that have little in common with laying a sympathetic hand on a patient's shoulder. Touch therapists, or, alternatively, "intuitive counselors," maintain that they can tap into a universal energy source and through their touch can transmit this energy to patients to achieve *healing*. Healing is often practiced by the physical "laying on" of the healer's hands onto the body of the patient. Most healers avoid actual contact: they keep their hands extended over the patient's body some inches above its surface. Others claim they do not even have to be in the patient's presence to achieve a therapeutic result. One common feature of all forms of healing is the belief that healing power lies in the healer rather than the patient. Those who believe that they have this power speak of using intuition to guide their hands around a patient's body, for the purpose of identifying energy blockage. Some believe in a form of cosmic energy associated with this talent, while others do not.

Although the scientific view provides little support for the energy aspects of therapeutic touch or healing, many individuals feel that healing has ameliorated problems that failed to respond to conventional medicine. Several critics have noted that healing is not so much about effecting cures as it is about increasing quality of life. Healers seem to work best with patients suffering from chronic and nonspecific complaints such as aches, pains, fatigue, and general distress. Not surprisingly, these are the very conditions that benefit from somatic awareness and associated musculoskeletal relaxation. Therapeutic touch is quite compatible with somatic awareness, as long as both patient and therapist understand that the positive sensations and feelings produced during sessions are generated *within* the patient *by* the patient. The touch therapist is able to facilitate these sensations and feelings by capitalizing on a strong human need for closeness, intimacy, and touch. Obviously, touching oneself in the same manner is not likely to produce comparable feelings, but patients can learn to reproduce the same feelings of well-being outside the touch session. In this way they are able to maintain, within conscious experience, those feelings of somatic well-being that are facilitated during the therapy sessions.

A number of therapists believe that they are more than facilitators of relaxation and self-soothing in their patients. Many believe that they are capable of identifying and releasing energy that they presume to be "stored" in the patient's body in some maladaptive fashion. CranioSacral therapists (Upledger, 1990) believe that they can identify, through touch, emotional conflict zones in the patient's body. They hold that negative bodily energy generated during previous emotional trauma is stored in the form of an "energy cyst" in the body. Energy enters the body and remains enclosed in the cyst, resulting in a disruption of normal bodily equilibrium. The CranioSacral therapist claims that through touch and body repositioning, he or she is able to establish an escape route for the trapped disruptive energy. The therapist claims to be able to measure the disruptive energy in a patient's body through electromyographic activity and also to sense the transfer of the disruptive energy from the patient's body to his/her own through the sensation of heat in his/her hands as they are passed over the trouble zones. CranioSacral medicine combines elements of physics, biomechanics, and psychoanalysis, but it does little to enhance a patient's understanding of how he or she might self-regulate the illness in question.

In spite of the dramatic "cures" that are often reported by those who believe in the healing power of their hands, including shamans and evangelical ministers, it would seem to be more advantageous to have people understand that they have even greater power within themselves to achieve health. Increasing one's level of somatic awareness may not be as dramatic as being "passed" by a healer, but it costs nothing and is as natural as the gentle breathing of air.

Energy Cardiology: The "Laying On of Heart"

The concept of healing energy has always been difficult to test through scientific research. This may change following the publication of a provocative paper by Russek and Schwartz (1996). They advanced the hypothesis that energy from the heart represents a model system of the health potential energy in health and illness. They use the term "energy" to signify any process that has "the ability to do work," and that can therefore influence other systems within the body, including atoms, molecules, cellular processes, physiological functioning, consciousness, and overt behavior:

> Of all the organs within the body, the heart is preeminent in terms of the centrality of its location, the richness of its connections to all the cells within the body, and particularly relevant here, the intensity of its energy transmission. This energy aspect of the heart does not receive much attention. But just as the heart not only pumps patterns of biochemical nutrients to every cell within the body through the circulation, it also "pumps" patterns of energy and information to every cell within the body through the circulation in the body. (p. 8)

The heart generates more than electrical energy with each cardiac cycle; it also generates magnetic energy, as well as sound, pressure, and thermal energies. Each of these different energy forms may convey different information to the individual.

Russek and Schwartz (1996) observed that the electrical potential from the heart, when compared to other biological generators within the body, is enormous. The electrical potential generated by the heart can be recorded from any site on the body. Thus, it follows that every cell in the body is "bathed" in the energy generated by the heart. Moreover, Russek and Schwartz believe that efforts should be made to understand the mixtures of types and frequencies of energy in different bodily units such as the heart and the brain.

Russek and Schwartz speculate that patterns of energies generated by the heart do not necessarily remain contained within the skin and that consequently *energies from one individual may interact with those of another individual* in the same vicinity:

> We must entertain the hypothesis that if two people are in the same room (though being in the same room is not required per se), patterns of cardiac energy travel between them, from Person A to Person B, and from Person B to Person A. Since both people are open dynamic systems, and since both people have functioning hearts, both people will generate cardiac energy patterns that extend into space, and these patterns may interact with one another in complex ways (even, in theory, when the people are separated by distance). (p. 13)

In mind–body medicine, it is typically assumed that consciousness influences the regulation of organ systems by neural mechanisms alone. But Russek and Schwartz believe that neural mechanisms may not be the only mechanisms by which consciousness regulates biological functioning. They suggest that consciousness affects the heart through the brain and peripheral nervous system, and that these modulated cardiac energy patterns have consequences both *within* and *between* persons. The heart—as bizarre as this may sound—*may* play a role in coordinating and integrating human health within and between individuals.

Russek and Schwartz are exploring their healing energy notions under the rubric of cardiac synchronized energy patterns, or CSEPs. They have conducted a series of experiments in which two people sit quietly opposite each other in the same room with their eyes closed, not communicating either visually, verbally, or kinesthetically. Electrocardiograms and electroencephalograms are recorded from both persons simultaneously. Russek and Schwartz believe that they will find evidence of heart energy emitted within persons as well as between persons:

> The strength of between-person CSEPs should vary as a function of distance (normally, force fields decrease in magnitude as the square of the distance increases). But it can also be varied by connecting people "elec-

trically." It is possible, for example, to create a between-person circuit. Using wires, person A's *left* hand can be connected to person B's *right* hand and person A's *right* hand to person B's *left* hand (an electric version of the mother and the fetus). When this is done, the magnitude of A's cardiac electrical potential will be observed strongly in person B's electrocardiogram, and vice versa—but the polarity will be reversed. . . . Such circuits occur naturally when people hold hands in this fashion, especially if their hands are moist, therefore making good electrical contact. (p. 17)

Russek and Schwartz speculate that the CSEP methodology provides a potentially powerful approach for addressing a whole host of basic science questions concerning the capacity of psychosocial factors to modulate energy patterns within and between individuals:

Does focused attention to the heart increase CSEPs within and between individuals? Does meditation (or sleep) allow the cells of the body to relax and synchronize more completely with cardiac energy? Do individual differences in variables such as personality and stress, imagery, and hypnotizability, and levels of emotional awareness and expression, modulate CSEPs within and between individuals? Do variables such as love and caring or anxiety and anger influence cardiac energy patterns within or between individuals? It is theoretically possible that the degree and complexity of interpersonal cardiac energy synchronization reflects levels of loving in caring relationships. Since individuals probably have unique CSEP signatures, it is possible that between-person CSEPs may show selective augmentation or reduction depending on the unique relationship. (p. 18)

The authors proposed that a good professional–patient relationship may, through empathy and caring, result in improved cardiac energy flow within the body and contribute to improvements in health. They also speculated that CSEPs may be at the basis of nonlocal healing. The term "nonlocal healing" refers to more than therapeutic touch; it encompasses a whole range of therapies and healing practices based on "moving energy" that specialists say they can feel even if their patients cannot. Nonlocal healing occurs when one person offers nonmaterial, nontouch help to another, and in the presence of the offer and the care the healee loses symptoms or becomes well (Cassidy, 1994).

The range of responses to the Russek and Schwartz's (1996) article reveals the diversity of thinking regarding alternative mind–body medicine. A cardiologist (Goldberger, 1996) questioned the logic of making the heart the center of a physiological universe, a cardiac version of the Ptolemaic system. This is extremely unlikely, he believes, given that the heart is under the control of the sinus node, which itself is driven by the autonomic nervous system. At the other end of the continuum are comments from energy healers who wholeheartedly agree with the hypotheses proposed. One healer who works with transplant patients follows the practice of putting her hands on the ice chest containing the explanted heart and reports receiving mental images that tell her how the heart feels both about the death of the donor and about the new body it is about to enter:

> A striking example of this occurred during a surgery in which the donated heart came from a woman who had been killed in an automobile accident. I knew that she was the daughter of the woman driving the car, but knew nothing more about the incident. When I put my hands over the heart, an image came to me of two women in the front seat of a car, arguing heatedly. I also got the message that the explanted heart now believed that if it got angry, it would be killed.
>
> When the heart was put into the patient's body, it would not beat in spite of all the chemicals that the concerned surgeon ordered the anesthesiologist to administer. I knew, from working with this patient beforehand, that she herself had a strong resistance to getting angry. Finally, when nothing the surgical team was doing seemed to be working, I leaned over and told the patient that she had to get angry, and to give the new heart permission to get angry—giving it the aggressive, forward-moving energy that I believe is the essence of that organ's life force. I held my hand above her heart and sent energy with the same message directly into the heart. Within half a minute it began to beat. When the surgery was over, the perfusionist (the technician who operates the heart–lung bypass machine) told me, "I don't know what you did, but I've never seen a heart come back so far or so fast." (Motz, 1996, p. 33)

In the opening chapter I reported that researchers at the Heartmath Institute have demonstrated that feeling appreciated is associated with energy changes in the electrocardiogram indicative of increased harmony of the sympathetic and parasympathetic innervation to the heart. The Chinese also attribute many positive human interpersonal qualities and experiences, including kindness, thoughtfulness, mercifulness, and generosity, to the heart. In fact, some Chinese would say that "if your heart is not good, then your entire person is not good" (Tung, 1994). Research that equivocally documents the within-person and between-person interactive effects of cardiac energy will be difficult to conduct. Moreover, such research, if successful, would not negate the fact that people still need to initiate, through their individual somatic awareness, the biological state needed for favorable cardiac energy transfers.

WHAT ABOUT BIOFEEDBACK?

Biofeedback (Schwartz & Associates, 1995) represents the most technical of the biobehavioral methods available for managing somatic symptoms. It involves the use of high-quality electronic instrumentation for measuring a number of physiological events, including sweat gland activity, blood pressure, skin temperature, respiration, and muscle activity. It is possible to receive certification through the Biofeedback Certification Institute of America (BCIA), whose program is designed to assure a level of quality control among practitioners.

Debate continues about what is actually being taught and learned during biofeedback training sessions. Patients are clearly *not* learning direct physiological control of the symptom in question. To a large extent, what they are learning is to relax in the presence of a supportive therapist. One might assume that biofeedback is synonymous with somatic awareness development. However, since somatic awareness is not an explicit goal of biofeedback practice, patients often fail to develop a generalized awareness of bodily well-being following a course of biofeedback therapy. Indeed, many patients come away from such therapy without developing any significant degree of somatic awareness.

The workhorse of the biofeedback field is electromyographic (EMG) feedback (Schwartz & Associates, 1995). The EMG is a complex measure of muscle activity obtained from recording electrodes placed on the skin. If a practitioner had to choose a single biofeedback modality to use across patients with different symptoms, his/her hands-down choice would be EMG biofeedback. EMG biofeedback has been successfully used with a wide variety of disorders and symptoms, including migraine and tension headache, chronic back pain, hypertension, incontinence, and diabetes (Schwartz & Associates, 1995).

The BCIA guidelines recommend that practitioners have skill with several biofeedback modalities, implying that different modalities are needed for different symptom circumstances. The position is debatable because the literature comparing different forms of biofeedback modalities and relaxation training across different disorders has not produced convincing results favoring one modality over the other.

Lehrer, Carr, Sargunaraj, and Woolfolk (1994) believe that unique physiological and clinical effects are associated with the various biofeedback and relaxation methods now in use. They reviewed a large number of studies that compared the effectiveness of the different techniques in controlling specific physiological systems and specific psychophysiological disorders. They found that EMG biofeedback was more effective than progressive relaxation in producing physiological effects during training sessions. However, the evidence that EMG biofeedback was more effective in controlling actual physiological symptoms was less than convincing. Another example provided in the Lehrer et al. review involved a comparison of thermal biofeedback with relaxation for the control of vascular symptoms such as Raynaud's disease, a psychophysiological condition that is associated with spasms in the blood vessels of the hands and feet. The goal of thermal biofeedback is to raise finger temperature with the purpose of increasing blood flow in the periphery. Lehrer et al. concluded that finger temperature biofeedback was more effective than relaxation training for Raynaud's. This may be the case, but the literature indicates that EMG biofeedback and/or relaxation are also effective in reducing Raynaud's symptoms.

Comparisons were made with other techniques, such as meditation, and with other disorders, such as migraine and muscle contraction headache. In each example Lehrer et al. make a weak case for using specific techniques for specific symptoms. In the case of migraine and muscle contraction headache, for example, they note that the evidence suggests that temperature training is more effective for migraine headache and EMG biofeedback is more effective for tension headache. At the same time they acknowledge that "both autonomic and muscular components exist in both types of headaches, and that improvement in headaches is not related to the degree of physiological control achieved" (p. 374). I believe that some common psychobiological processes are being altered across different headache disorders (Bakal et al., 1994), and that these processes can be altered with or without biofeedback training. The processes likely involve alterations in subtle musculoskeletal activity in the head, neck, and shoulder regions. The alteration of this musculoskeletal activity through biofeedback, if it is to be used, is best addressed through EMG feedback. However, the practice of EMG biofeedback, although definitely useful in clinical practice, is not necessary to achieve somatic awareness.

Biofeedback training is often perceived by patients as a high-powered technique that is applied to them as opposed to a technique that guides their discovery of somatic awareness. People who undergo biofeedback may see it as an intervention much like massage, transcutaneous electrical nerve stimulation (TENS), or acupuncture, procedures wherein something viewed as mysterious but presumably curative *is done* to their body. Biofeedback specialists do little to challenge this perception; indeed, they often deliberately take steps to ensure that their intervention is understood by the patient as a highly technical and professional intervention. An examination of the criteria for training as a biofeedback therapist reinforce the notion that there are exact skills and knowledge involved that make professional intervention mandatory. For example, the following capabilities are listed as essential:

1. Training, knowledge, experience, and skill with a variety of non-instrumentation-based physiological self-regulatory procedures.
2. Training, knowledge, experience, and skill with at least a few biofeedback modalities, including at least electromyographic (EMG), temperature, and electrodermal biofeedback.
3. Training, knowledge, experience, and skill with other modalities such as pulse, breathing, and/or electroencephalographic (EEG) biofeedback. (Schwartz, 1995, p. 245)

I agree with the need for professional training and competence in the use of biofeedback. However, these required attributes deal solely with technical skill. Although "good verbal skills" and other personal attributes are deemed desirable, there is no guarantee that following such training an individual therapist will be adept at recognizing and reinforcing patient acquisition of somatic awareness. Similarly, there is no guarantee that following a course of therapy with a trained therapist, a patient will recognize the bodily sensations needed to prevent the occurrence of the symptom in his/her day-to-day living. Patients who receive biofeedback training do not necessarily improve in their general level of somatic awareness, and consequently do not necessarily exhibit significant and/or lasting symptom improvement.

It may seem odd and paradoxical to suggest that biofeedback is not necessarily associated with increased somatic awareness and reliable symptom management. After all, biofeedback, once discovered, was hailed as a means of using the mind to control the body. However, I need to reiterate that psychobiological disorders like migraine are very complicated conditions, not just at the physiological level but also at the psychological level. Biofeedback transducers placed on the skin, regardless of the nature of the modality used (EMG, temperature, EEG), cannot be expected, when presented as a means of attaining "physiological control," to reflect this complexity.

During the early years of my clinical use of EMG biofeedback for treating migraine and tension headache, it became evident to me that although patients often enjoyed the somatic sensations accompanying relaxing of muscle groups during training sessions, they had great difficulty experiencing and then maintaining similar bodily sensations outside the training sessions. They also seemed to benefit as much if not more from our discussion and the fact that *someone was willing to lis-*

ten to them talk about their headache. I recall a session with a patient in which the EMG biofeedback device would not work. Rather than cancel the session, I spoke to the patient about his life, past and present. At the end of our time together, I apologized for the technical problem with the equipment and the patient replied "Don't apologize—this has been our best session yet!" Therapists know, however, that such positive ventilatory experiences are seldom sufficient to promote relief from headache. The patient still needs to acquire and maintain an inner sense of bodily relaxation.

EMG biofeedback can be very useful for helping therapists and patients identify elevated tension and develop strategies for altering tension in specific body regions (e.g., chest, jaw, neck, shoulders), but it is too narrow in emphasis to be used as the sole means of enhancing somatic awareness. Patients need to incorporate their biofeedback experiences into their day-to-day living before true therapeutic change will occur. In this respect, biofeedback is no different than many of the other alternative therapies currently available. For example, patients who receive massage therapy often feel extremely relaxed and symptom-free immediately following the session but lose awareness of this positive bodily state within hours of resuming normal living. People must learn to relate their somatic experiences attained in the clinic to their somatic experiences during daily living.

In the halcyon days of biofeedback, EEG alpha training was used to achieve a state of consciousness some equated with a "natural high." This "high" was eventually attributed to demand characteristics of the situation and subject expectations rather than to the actual EEG state. Alpha training was abandoned in favor of less costly relaxation training. Although we are not normally aware of our brain wave activity, EEG feedback has resurfaced under the guise of *EEG neurofeedback.* Originally designed to assist with attention deficit disorder in children, EEG neurofeedback is now being used to treat chronic pain, migraine, anxiety, and other somatic symptoms. Proponents are once again making great claims for its effectiveness, but it is questionable that brainwave retraining is actually taking place during the biofeedback sessions. We have seen a number of patients who, when taking EEG neurofeedback sessions on a daily basis, felt less anxiety and pain, but who experienced a full return of the symptoms within days of discontinuing treatment. They had learned nothing about how to recognize and manage bodily sensations outside of the clinical sessions. It would seem to make better sense to place less emphasis on "brain training" clinics and more emphasis on having people get in touch with the somatic aspect of their being.

EFFORTLESS BREATHING

Experiencing bodily well-being depends on a particular style of breathing. In fact, the way people breathe may determine their ability to utilize somatic awareness for healing. Breathing may be the cornerstone of the sensations we experience as overall bodily well-being. The connection between breathing and health is universally recognized. For example, breathing retraining continues to serve as the foundation for most biobehavioral interventions and alternative therapies. Also, gestalt therapists recommend that all health professionals, in conducting a clinical assessment, should make a visual determination of the client/patient's breathing patterns during the interview, both in response to neutral issues and in response to emotional and stressful issues.

Recognition of the relationship between breathing and mental health is found in Carl Jung's (1875–1961) individuation concept. Jung postulated that the collective unconscious has a natural tendency of striving toward psychological wholeness. This natural striving or growth process involves the recognition in consciousness of tendencies reflecting the opposite sex. Males harbor a "feminine" tendency, called by Jung the *anima*, and females harbor a masculine tendency, called by Jung the *animus*. Anima is Latin for "soul" or "breath," while *animus* means "mind" in Latin. In both men and women, the sensations of breathing are associated with feeling attributes involving nurture, tenderness, softness, and grace. Thus, taking control of one's body through breathing constitutes a Jungian form of feminism. At a more general level, it means coming to accept, explore, and care for the body that is ours.

Breathing is vital to developing somatic awareness as it is the only bodily process which is under both automatic and conscious bodily control. Patel (1994) characterized the bidirectional relationship which exists between breathing and psychological states as follows:

> [Breathing] affects the way we think and feel, the quality of what we create, and how we function in our daily life. Breathing affects our psychological and physiological states, while our psychological states affect the pattern of our breathing. For example, when anxious, we tend to hold our breath and speak at the end of inspiration in a high-pitched voice. Depressed people tend to sigh and speak at the end of expiration in a low-toned voice. A child having a temper tantrum holds his or her breath until blue in the face. Hyperventilation causes not only anxiety but also such a variety of symptoms that patients can go from one specialty department to another until a wise clinician spots the abnormal breathing pattern and the patient is trained to shift from maladaptive to normal breathing behavior. (p. ix)

Some readers might feel that breathing is so straightforward there is nothing significant to learn by paying attention to the process—inhaling, exhaling, and inhaling again is no big deal. In terms of developing somatic awareness, however, breathing, especially effortless breathing is a very big deal. Breathing should be slow and involve the diaphragm but even more important it should occur *without effort.*

The Muscles and Mechanics of Normal Breathing

Breathing is a highly individualized action and varies tremendously from one individual to the next. Breathing is also intricately related to metabolic functions, speech, emotion, and even personality. "Normal" breathing, then, is not simply a mechanical state that can be readily described or measured independent of situational demands and/or other characteristics of the person. It is possible, however, to characterize a generally optimal breathing pattern, albeit each individual might experience this pattern in his/her own unique way. For a description of the muscles and mechanics of breathing, we rely on an article by Naifeh (1994), to which the reader is referred for more detail.

During normal breathing the chest rises and falls and the abdominal area moves outward and inward. Two sets of primary muscles control these movements ("primary" is a term used to emphasize that these muscles are the only ones used under normal conditions). These muscles are the external intercostal (rib cage) muscles beneath the ribs and the diaphragm, which separates the thorax, containing the heart and lungs, from the abdominal cavity. The intercostals lift the ribs up and out and are responsible for thoracic or chest breathing. The movement of the ribcage upward and outward causes a negative pressure in the lungs that is equalized by air moving into the lungs, inflating them during the inspiration phase of breathing:

Now to simplify this discussion of lung inflation somewhat, let us first consider the analogy of blowing up a balloon. There are two ways to inflate a balloon; one is to blow air into it by some means. To do this we have to raise the pressure of the air with which we are going to inflate the balloon so that it will flow into the balloon, because initially the air inside the balloon is at the same pressure as the earth's atmosphere. . . . There is, however, another way to inflate the balloon. If we place the balloon inside a chamber so that only its neck sticks out, and the chamber is sealed around the neck, then the inside of the balloon will be connected to the atmosphere, but the inside of chamber (which surrounds the outside of the balloon) will not. If we then create a vacuum inside the chamber, the pressure around the outside of the balloon will be less than that on the inside of the balloon, which is still equal to the atmospheric pressure. The greater pressure inside the balloon will cause it to expand, and its expansion will increase its volume. This, in turn, will cause the pressure inside the balloon to drop, because the same amount of air is contained in a larger space. The drop in pressure will cause more air from the atmosphere to flow into the balloon. . . . In a similar way, our respiratory muscles increase and decrease a vacuum in the chest cavity around our lungs in order to produce inspiration and expiration. The chest and lungs are designed so that there is a negative pressure, or vacuum, in the space between the lungs and chest wall (the intrapleural space). This vacuum creates a suction force, which holds the lungs tightly against the chest wall. Therefore, when the chest cavity expands because the inspiratory muscles pull the ribs up and out, the lungs enlarge also, still being held tightly against the chest wall by the suction force. Now, because the lungs expand, the pressure of air inside them decreases, becoming lower than the atmospheric pressure; more air flows in from the atmosphere in order to equalize the pressure between the lungs and outer environment. And thus inspiration occurs. Expiration is essentially all this going backwards. When the chest wall goes back to its expiratory position, the chest cavity becomes a smaller container again; this allows the lungs to partially deflate because there is less of a vacuum. The extra air they acquired during inspiration is now filling a smaller space, so the pressure inside the lungs goes up. This forces air to flow out of the lungs until the pressure inside the lungs is again equal to the pressure in the atmosphere. . . . Contraction of the diaphragm produces inspiration through identical mechanisms. (pp. 23–24)

Eastern and Western Breathing

In Eastern cultures, breathing is central to a number of religious or quasi-religious exercises advocated for facilitating spiritual and physical health. In China, *qi gong* is a form of exercise that combines graceful movements and deep breathing as a means of "blowing and respiring, getting rid of the stale and taking in the fresh." *Qi* (sometimes spelled "chi") means vital energy, vital essence, or vital breath. When one is feeling well, then *qi* flows through the body smoothly. Tai chi integrates breathing with exercise, meditation, and martial arts. In tai chi circular exercise movements are designed to balance and strengthen the chi and thereby prevent illness. During practice, the mind is concentrated on the *tan tien,* a point two inches below the navel. The beauty of these exercises lies not in the abdominal breathing per se but in the graceful body movements such as those associated with strumming a lute or imitating a crane skimming over water.

The best known of the meditative methods for training breathing comes from the set of practices called hatha yoga. In Sanskrit *yoga* means "yoking," which has to do with preparing the individual for joining with God. The preparation for a life of hatha yoga is demanding and requires the completion of a series of increasingly difficult skills. The initial stages deal with "cleansing" of the mind in the form of developing restraint and obedience. Next comes practice in the asana postures, which are ways of sitting or holding positions for long periods of time. The fourth stage is the pranayama or breath control, which is designed to generate a stable breathing pattern and relax the body.

The pranayama technique consists of three separate breathing components: (1) slowing and regularizing the breath by prolonging the expiratory phase, (2) increasing diaphragmatic breathing, and (3) adding resistance to each breath (Chandra, 1994). Expiration is prolonged to twice the duration of inspiration in order to induce mental and physical relaxation. Resistance is added in a number of ways, one of which involves alternating occlusion between the left and right nostrils. It is assumed that there are important connections between the nasal passages and the individual's mental state:

> During spontaneous breathing, inhaling through the left nostril is said by most people to have a calming, beneficial, stabilizing effect, while breathing through the right nostril is destabilizing, and ultimately enervating. A balance between the two modes is thought to be most suitable for the challenges of daily life, and is put forth as a teleological explanation for the ultradian rhythm of congestion/decongestion that occurs in the nose throughout the day. This cycle of naturally occurring congestion in one nostril with relative decongestion in the other nostril, followed by the reverse, occurs every 1½–4 hours and has been described by yogic practitioners for hundreds of years. (p. 223)

Western approaches to breathing lack the religious heritage associated with tai chi and yoga. Orthodox followers of the Eastern techniques might well view Western breathing retraining in isolation from spirituality retraining as being very superficial in approach. However, living in the West, in the absence of a guiding religion, makes Eastern breathing exercises difficult to practice and even more difficult to incorporate into daily self-experiences. For example, try paying attention to your nostril airflow while reading this page.

Benson and colleagues (Benson, Beary, & Carol, 1974) recognized that it is difficult to teach mystical strategies to nonmystics, that is, people living in the West. To solve this problem, they devised a form of meditative breathing more compatible with our "fast-food" way of thinking and behaving. They called the technique the *relaxation response* and hypothesized that with regular practice it is possible to produce a hypometabolic bodily state comparable to what has been claimed for transcendental meditation. The technique is practiced by sitting quietly with eyes closed and breathing out through your nose. With each outward breath, you are to say the word "one" silently to yourself. The word "one" serves as a mantra that facilitates the maintenance of a passive attitude. Scientific support for the belief that this "response" is more powerful than straightforward relaxation has not been provided. Furthermore, the procedure still requires stepping outside of regular thought and behavior to practice.

Some therapists continue to use breathing as a link to the unconscious. They believe that it is possible to get at the root of psychological and bodily tension. Both bioenergetic and gestalt therapists employ special exercises to link breathing to repressed feelings. A patient with tight jaw muscles, for example, might be asked to breathe deeply and "growl" whenever he/she becomes aware of clenching his/her teeth. In this way angry feelings are made more salient and manageable. The assumption is that repressed feelings must be identified and released before breathing can normalize. These therapists owe their techniques to Wilhelm Reich (1942) who in his studies of muscle tone found breathing disturbances in virtually all of the patients he treated. He developed *vegetotherapy* (the term "vegetative" refers to the involuntary nature of the autonomic nervous system) to deal with the impact of unconscious impulses on internal bodily rhythms of the body involving the beating of the heart, secretions from glands, and peristalsis of the gut. He believed that disturbed breathing patterns were the root cause of disturbances in these internal rhythms.

Reich developed special exercises designed to release repressed emotions and normalize breathing. Reich described *muscle-bound or militaristic* breathing as a stiffening of the chest muscles and tightening of the rib cage, with an accompanying reduction in the mobility of the diaphragm. During breathing the chest remains raised and overcontrolled. The stiffness of the rib intercostal muscles, the chest pectorals, and the shoulder deltoids was taken as a sign of self-control and restraint. The pulled-back shoulders literally express *holding back* (Boadella, 1994).

Stress management therapists have also noted a high incidence of *collarbone breathing* in their clients/patients (Timmons, 1994). For many years the educational system encouraged a similar breathing pattern through the posture edict "stomach in, shoulders back, and chest out." Such a pattern may have positive benefits for the outer body image but can lead to suffocation of the inner somatic self. An extreme breathing pattern common to many patients with anxiety and breathing disorders is called *paradoxical* breathing. In this form of breathing, the direction of movement in the chest and abdomen are in opposition to each other. When the chest expands, the abdomen goes in and vice versa. Inspiration is associated with an upward (rather than outward) movement of the chest and a "sucking in" of the belly. Diaphragmatic movements are out of touch with movements of the chest. Children with severe asthma attacks also show this pattern of breathing, but it is not known whether they exhibit paradoxical breathing outside the asthma episode.

In Germany a number of schools of therapy deal specifically with the mechanics of breathing. These schools had their origins in the work of Elsa Gindler and her disciples, who believe that human beings are alienated from their natural inner somatic self (Buchholz, 1994). Gindler and her followers believe that too much emphasis is put on training the outer muscles while the deeper muscular layers and skeletal muscles that contribute to natural uprightness and effortless breathing are ignored. They use the concept of *eutonie* to describe a form of somatic awareness based on breathing movement characterized by flexibility and readiness to react to changing demands. Buchholz argued that eutonus is controlled by the gamma nervous system, a distinct information system within the muscle tissue and linked to CNS structures involved with breathing. According to Gindler and her followers, the gamma nervous system can be activated through somatic awareness, touch, and subtle movements. Although it is not clear which nervous system attributes are subsumed under the gamma label, it is significant that bodily systems specific to awareness of healthy breathing are hypothesized to exist.

There are many breathing retraining scripts available, all of which encourage a healthier coordination of the abdominal, intercostal, chest, neck and shoulder muscles. To determine what kind of breather a patient is (chest or belly), therapists will ask the patient to place one hand on the chest and the other hand on the stomach. Chest breathers will notice that upon breathing in, their chest will expand and their shoulders will rise, while their stomach does not move or moves inward. Belly breathers, on the other hand, will show little or no movement of the chest and shoulders when they inhale. Instead, their stomach will move outward with inhalation and inward with exhalation.

Breathing retraining is far from straightforward. In all instances it should be implemented with a sense of understanding of how the patient usually breathes. Timmons (1994) cautioned against the indiscriminate application of breathing retraining techniques. She approvingly quoted L. C. Lum: "It is better not to change a patient's breathing unless you know what you are doing" (p. 276). Physical therapists believe that breathing retraining of patient populations should be done only by those with knowledge of the anatomy and mechanics of respiratory disorders and diseases. Fried (1993) cautioned that persons with seemingly functional breathing disorders may be suffering from metabolic disorders caused by serious medical illness. Thus, a medical examination should also be conducted to determine that behavioral alteration of breathing is not contraindicated.

Once a patient is deemed suitable from a medical perspective for breathing retraining, it is necessary to appreciate the patient's individualistic way of breathing and the complex psychobiological processes that are contributing to breathing under different circumstances. Today we are only beginning to recognize how individualistic breathing patterns are. In the opening chapter I discussed how women in active childbirth labor differ in terms of their thoughts, feelings, and breathing rates. During childbirth training, women are shown how to utilize a pattern of slow and deep breathing during early or latent labor and to accentuate this pattern with the onset of contractions. The assumption is that this breathing pattern will reduce pain and distress and facilitate bodily relaxation. However, no group data demonstrate that women are actually able to achieve this pattern once the action begins. In pilot observations of 14 women who had received training in breathing, only 6 were able to reduce their breathing rate and increase their depth of breathing during latent labor (Hesson, Hill, & Bakal, 1997). Even within this small group there was enormous variability in the degree of change in the two respiratory parameters. Increases in volume ranged from 42 ml to 1,642 ml, while reductions in breathing rate ranged from 0.5 cycles per minute to 7.3 cycles per minute. The remaining women showed responses in one or both measures opposite from the direction in which they were trained.

There is no strong evidence that maladaptive breathing patterns are readily *normalized*. Critics of recipe approaches to breathing in childbirth have likewise argued that artificial breathing techniques may actually inhibit maternal relaxation when individual differences in characteristic respiratory parameters are ignored. There is some evidence that having these individuals change their characteristic way of breathing is far from a simple matter. Gallego and Perruchet (1991) observed that with some individuals the adoption of an artificial breathing pattern resulted in breathing irregularity. In clinical situations patients have often breathed in a specific way for a good portion of their lives. For example, patients with anxiety-based somatic symptoms are often thoracic breathers and have difficulty understanding and breathing in any other fashion. This difficulty can become pronounced if they are instructed with technique-oriented interventions aimed at altering their preferred way of breathing. Many patients with respiratory disorders/diseases who have received formal instruction in breathing still do not know how to experience a relaxed breath. They often try to mimic a pattern of "deep breathing" suggested by a therapist but invariably they continue to exaggerate their preferred way of breathing by expanding and raising their chest and shoulders. They seldom feel better for breathing this way. Elderly patients who have breathed primarily with the chest all their lives find instruction in abdominal breathing confusing and at times hyperventilate as they try to follow the instructions they are provided.

The solution to advising patients who are breathing in an effortful fashion is to encourage them to breathe effortlessly. Most patient can follow instructions to breathe effortlessly easier than they can follow some suggestion to take a deep breath. They often interpret the suggestion as simply breathing *naturally* or *normally*—which for different patients means different things in terms of actual breathing style. For some, it means that the chest muscles are more relaxed, which results in both the chest and abdomen moving outward and inward together. For others, it will mean a shift to largely abdominal breathing. Most patients, with direction, can identify a pattern of breathing that is comfortable for them. This pattern is generally associated with pleasant sensations, relaxation of the chest muscles, and improved synchrony of the thorax and abdomen during inspiration and expiration.

By encouraging patients to relate their breathing to a natural relaxed pattern, we can help them to better connect each breath cycle to ongoing thoughts, feelings, and bodily sensations associated with somatic well-being. This is important because if they are left to exercises and recipe-type instructions, they are prone to hyperventilate if they try to implement the exercise during a period of heightened anxiety or fear.

ON "LETTING GO"

Therapists who work with biofeedback, breathing retraining, and other self-regulatory strategies are all familiar with the patient complaint "I have tried that technique and it doesn't work." Usually the difference between patients who succeed and patients who fail can be expressed in terms of letting go: some can let go and some cannot let go. The phrase "letting go" appears very frequently in the bodily self-control literature. It can refer to quite different levels of abstraction. For example, it can refer to letting go of nongratifying relationships, negative feelings of hostility and anger, an unwillingness to forgive, guilt, a relentless pursuit of perfectionism and so forth. It can also refer to somatic awareness. In my use of the phrase, "letting go" represents a clinical heuristic for achieving bodily control without effort. Given the systemic nature of human functioning, an individual generally needs to let go at multiple levels in order to achieve health.

In a classic paper on letting go and anxiety, Heide and Borkovec (1984) observed that while procedures such as deep breathing can reduce subjective anxiety and physiological hyperactivity, the same procedures in some individuals and under some circumstances can *increase* anxiety. They discussed in detail a number of psychological processes that contribute to relaxation-induced anxiety, the most important of which is a fear of letting go combined with an attempt to maintain relaxation through active, effortful strategies. "Control can be defined as the ability to modify outcomes by voluntary responding . . . ; it refers to the individual's capacity to affect the world. Effort, in contrast, refers to active or applied force; it concerns the intensity of the individual's active demands to affect the world" (p. 3).

Active effort usually works best in coping with demands external to oneself and *not* with regulating bodily processes that are largely involuntary in nature. A common admonition in relaxation/biofeedback training, for example, is "You cannot *force* yourself to relax, you must *allow* yourself to relax." Effort, because of its association with musculoskeletal force, is generally counterproductive in trying to bring under control bodily processes that by nature are involuntary. I discussed earlier how using effort to control breathing can often be countertherapeutic. Control of breathing, or any other bodily function, is best achieved through effortless control.

Letting go, at the bodily level, can be both specific and nonspecific in form. The phenomenological experience associated with letting go is observed in all relaxation/biofeedback techniques. When elicited in the context of clinical symptoms, the patient's immediate experience is often one of symptom reduction or even symptom disappearance. My first observation of the potential power of this psychobiological state occurred some 20 years ago during the routine application of forehead EMG biofeedback training for headache. During their training sessions, some patients would show a sudden and spontaneous lowering of EMG activity. This sudden decrease was experienced as total relaxation in the body region underneath the recording electrodes. Unfortunately, the state was often transient and not readily identified by the patients. I suspect that the sudden reduction in EMG activity and accompanying feelings of tension release are the psychobiological equivalent of localized letting go. Similar experiences have been reported by patients suffering from hypertension, chest pain, gastrointestinal distress, back pain, asthma, and arthritis.

People who are used to exerting themselves to solve life's external problems, especially those people with exacting standards for themselves and others, will find the idea of letting go and soothing oneself as a form of "giving up." They may find the new bodily awareness as unnatural and anxiety-provoking. Wegner and colleagues (Wegner, Broome, & Blumberg, 1997) developed a theory of *ironic processes of mental control* to explain the paradoxical effects that may occur in some individuals who make intentional efforts to let go. Mental control succeeds, and also fails, as a result of the function of two processes of mental control that fluctuate in their influence on the mind. The *intentional operating process* searches for mental contents consistent with the desired state of mind—in the case of letting go, relaxing thoughts or images, or soothing bodily sensations. Accompanying this is an *ironic monitoring process* that searches for mental contents that indicate a failure or fear of the desired state of mind. The ironic monitor leads to thoughts indicating a failure to relax and might include arousing or stressful thoughts and images, as well as bodily sensations of arousal.

The operating and monitoring processes normally work together to provide the kind of mental control necessary for relaxation, sleep, and the like. However, when stress, worry, or anxiety impinge on the mind, not only is the operating process undermined but the ironic monitoring process may also be unleashed to activate the very anxiety-producing thoughts, feelings, and sensations that one is trying so hard to control. Thus intentional control to let go under stress might result in the opposite of the intended state. Many patients who report trying to relax are quick to describe their failure and rejection of the effort.

A life history characterized by physical and/or sexual abuse can often lead to the opposite intended state of letting go. Traumatized individuals have special difficulty letting go, presumably for fear of losing bodily and mental control. A dramatic example of the initial negative consequences of letting go in a sexually abused patient occurred during a routine EMG training session. The patient was a young female who was referred to me for biofeedback to assist with the management of severe neck and shoulder pain. Her shoulder muscles were in a state of heightened muscle tension that prevented her from turning her head more than a few degrees. No mention was made in the referral or by the patient herself of a previous history of sexual abuse.

During the initial biofeedback session, EMG electrodes were attached to her right shoulder and she was instructed to relax and let go in whatever way she could. After a few minutes, the EMG activity suddenly fell from extremely high levels to near zero. The patient reported severe sharp and stabbing pain in her head and appeared to lose consciousness. Given the dramatic fall in EMG activity, it appeared that the EMG machine was malfunctioning. But palpation of the patient's shoulder while she was in an almost trancelike state revealed that her shoulder muscles were completely relaxed. As she regained normal "consciousness," the EMG activity slowly returned to above-normal levels. The patient had previously experienced the same loss of consciousness while attending a neurology clinic. The attending neurologist determined that her EEG during this period was indicative of consciousness rather than of unconsciousness. We were to discover in later sessions that this patient had experienced a history of severe sexual abuse that contributed both to the dramatic tension levels and the reluctance to allow her body to relax. Still, the potential for bodily letting go remained within her as demonstrated by the sudden, albeit temporary, release of tension in her shoulder muscles. Many treatment sessions were required before she could allow herself to let go in a natural fashion without being overwhelmed by thoughts and feelings associated with the earlier abuse. She has since become a nurse and now incorporates somatic awareness into her professional and personal life.

The objective in encouraging letting go is to teach patients to recognize the psychological and bodily states that interfere with positive somatic awareness experiences. The clinician who encourages the patient to let go needs to appreciate the psychobiological nature of this heuristic. Often letting go at the bodily level cannot occur until letting go takes place in the mind, either consciously or unconsciously. I provided examples of how lifestyle demands compete for bodily attention and make it difficult to let go. But I also provided examples of individuals who let go of self-criticism and self-destructive lifestyles in search of inner bodily health. There are many different levels of the letting go heuristic that need to be fostered. The benchmark for determining how much change is required is how successful the patient is in working toward maintaining a healthy bodily self. Many patients can attain a high degree of symptom/illness management with minor adjustments in their personal cognitive coping styles, work habits, and/or living arrangements. Other patients, however, are required to make more drastic changes within themselves and their environments before they can attain bodily well-being. Healthy somatic awareness can be achieved in many different ways, from monitoring breathing and bodily sensations, to releasing the need to be important or to be loved by everyone. Our Buddha can be discovered in many different ways.

INTEGRATING SOMATIC AWARENESS
INTO PROFESSIONAL PRACTICE

The utilization of somatic awareness as a health care universal requires that health professionals become comfortable with accepting and working with patient reports of positive as well as negative bodily experiences. Somatic awareness is a natural dimension of human functioning and can be utilized by any professional working with patients. Health professionals from all disciplines have the means to make a quantum advance in their ability to integrate the various dimensions of human health within their practice. Moreover, health professionals come from a variety of different intellectual backgrounds and this very diversity of educational/training experience has the potential to add new practice ideas in the use of somatic awareness.

Somatic awareness can constitute the clinical principle required to establish a truly holistic practice of health care:

> Treatment becomes, in the holistic model, not one of "cure" or "pallia-tion," but one of facilitating bodily modification in a context of increased [self and body] awareness. Thus, practitioners generally see themselves as facilitating the patient's own healing rather than "doing" it for the patient. The practitioner is still an authority, but this time not in hierar-chy with the patient so much as in partnership. The practitioner has spe-cialty knowledge, but only the patient can exert knowledge of his/her own body and the context of his/her life. Thus, the practitioner is expected to guide the patient, and the patient is expected to take responsi-bility by learning to listen to his or her own body and then applying the resulting new information to living so as to avoid future illness and adapt to existing limitations. Also, because holistic practitioners see themselves as essentially entering the life space of the patient, they are usually at pains to be gentle and caring. They consider the behaviors to be them-selves healing (Cassidy, 1994, p. 15)

Intellectually, health professionals accept the idea that most patients with chronic illness conditions require a biopsychosocial understanding. During clinical practice, however, they may find that treating a patient within the context of such a broad framework is diffi-cult to do. Physicians faced with patients who are suffering from chronic pain or who cannot sleep may well recognize that the patient has ongoing difficulties with anxiety, depression, and marriage. But rather than attempting to manage all these issues themselves, they find it more convenient to prescribe an analgesic or a sedative and then refer the patient to other professionals more appropriately trained. Thus, for medical professionals in particular, the phrase "holistic health" still implies an "adding on" of the psychosocial aspects of health and illness to existing biomedicine rather than working within a truly integrated framework. It is not surprising, given this approach, that patients themselves have difficulty grasping the holistic aspects of their condition.

If one listens attentively to multidisciplinary team discussions of patient problems, one cannot help but notice how fragmented the understanding and management of a patient can be. Each professional sees the patients only from his/her perspective. These different perspectives do not necessarily complement one another. The cause of chronic pain in the elderly patient may be attributed to osteoarthritis, depression, bad posture, tension, lack of exercise, diet, loneliness, or all of the above and more, depending on how many different professionals take part in the discussion. Each professional assesses the patient from a specific disciplinary perspective and makes treatment recommendations within the boundaries of his/her discipline's knowledge base. The patient may be advised, by successive professionals, to use more analgesic medication, less analgesic medication, a different medication or no medication; to change diet; to relax or to exercise; to wear different shoes; to avoid thoughts of pain; to stay out of bed or to stay in bed; to attend marital therapy; to change living arrangements; and so forth, depending on how many team members are involved.

Clearly, there is a wellness benefit to health professionals not only providing valuable discipline-specific expertise, but also sharing enough common ground in holistic health practice to treat patients. Somatic awareness is ideally suited for establishing a common perspective for guiding the various interventions of a multidisciplinary health care team. Physician members of the team, for example, need to alleviate patient fears regarding undetected organic causes for their complaints and provide the patient with the understanding that self-regulation and management rather than cure is called for. This determination also gives the other members of the health care team the freedom to bring to bear their specific therapeutic strategies for managing the illness condition.

Once the allied professionals are called upon, there is much they can do, within their own discipline-specific perspective, to enhance patient development of somatic awareness during the rehabilitation process. Let's take chronic pain as an example. Physiotherapists employ techniques such as gentle stretch, heat, massage, and hydrotherapy to improve the patient's bodily well-being. Nurses intuitively understand the importance of calming the patient in pain. They know that the gentle application of a salve to a painful arthritic knee is often more effective than an analgesic. They also know that a glass of warm milk and a shared moment with a patient who cannot sleep is more comforting than a sleeping pill. Recreational therapists know how to tap somatic awareness through reading, listening to music, singing, and a host of other leisure activities. As these few examples indicate, there is much that can done when all efforts are directed toward enhancing somatic awareness. For all members of the therapeutic team, it becomes more rewarding to share a patient's bodily experiences with an illness than to attempt to reduce the illness to objective observations alone.

All health professionals should maintain a high level of empathy for the patient. In this way the patient knows that it is okay to listen to his/her body, to connect bodily sensations to feelings, and to report these linkages to the therapist.

> The healer's ability to selectively acknowledge a patient's emotional, psychological experiences enables the patient to become more aware of his or her own inner states and their implicit messages for action and change—perhaps, in turn, activating the multiple pathways of biopsychosocial processes required for self-regulation. . . . Healers selectively acknowledge a patient's inner experience by observing many levels of emotional and biobehavioral responses and then reflecting back core information to the patient in both verbal and nonverbal ways. In essence, healers act as naturalistic biofeedback systems, selectively amplifying emotional awareness in a person who is repressed, and containing such awareness in the case of a person flooded with affective overload. (Dafter, 1996, p. 69)

Matthews, Suchman, and Branch (1993) took the issue of empathy a step further and described the importance of making "connexions" with patients. Connexions are those quasi-spiritual moments in the physician–patient encounter marked by "a physiologic reaction, such as gooseflesh or a chill; by an immediacy of awareness of the patient's situation . . . ; by a sense of being part of a larger whole; and by a lingering feeling of joy, peacefulness or awe" (p. 973). These mental expectations might be a bit difficult to elicit throughout the day, patient after patient. However, Matthews et al. understand the importance of using communication strategies that allow patients to tell their story.

The therapeutic use of somatic awareness is achieved by listening to patients talk about their symptom not just in terms of sickness or illness but in terms of what the symptom means to the patient, what the patient does to bring the symptom on, and—most importantly—what the patient can do to lessen or eliminate the symptom. Most patients with chronic symptom conditions can describe thoughts, feelings, and behaviors that they do that will significantly improve their condition, at least for the moment. These activities include resting, walking, visualizing pleasant imagery, having a bath, sipping tea, reading, and sleeping. Activities that patients use on their own to generate feelings of bodily well-being need to be identified and strengthened. Most patients also recognize specific fears and concerns that worsen their symptom presentation. They do not expect their physicians or other health professionals to fix all of their problems.

Professionals working with somatic awareness need to be careful not to lose sight of the central objective in working with a patient. During a clinical interview it is important to integrate the patient's symptom or illness with his/her personal life but at the same time not to automatically reinterpret the symptom as a direct manifestation of some unresolved psychological state, conflict, personality disorder, or unhappy living arrangement. Past and present life events are part of the context in which a patient experiences and copes with illness, but we should be cautious in overly interpreting the significance of such events. We can examine this issue using excerpts from a physician–patient interview.

The interview is taken from an article discussing the value of listening to the words patients use to better understand the relation their symptoms and illness have to their personal life (Katz & Shotter, 1996). Although the narrative below refers to a physician–patient interview, the material is relevant to all health professionals. The authors make a valid case for appreciating the cultural view in which patients experience and describe their bodies and illnesses:

> If we privilege the medical voice alone, then what the patient says is located in the body, selectively translated into medical language, and the rest set aside; that is, issues to do with cultural and social processes become marginalized. However, if we care to notice other features of the talk in such interviews—not only of the patient but of the doctor too—its tone, its emotional richness or emptiness, its nuance and variation, the rhythm of the speech used, whether it is monotonic and formulaic, whether it is empathic or wondering talk, full of feeling, varying in tone and intensity, whether the person themselves talks, or describes others, in first-person or third-person language, then we can find something else besides symptoms of disease in the interview talk. It is in our capacity to respond to these fleeting moments in extraordinary, rather than ordinary, routine ways that enables us to create a novel form of living contact with them. For it is in those living moments of talk that we can find the patient, their "world," and what it is like for them, trying in the face of their illness, to live in it. (p. 921)

The example provided concerns a Haitian woman who presents to the medical resident with chest and gynecological symptoms. In the following passage the doctor is designated as "D" and the patient as "B":

D began by asking B:
"How old are you?"
"33."
"What brought you to the primary Care Clinic?", D asked.
"Oh 2 months ago, I was coughing, deep in my stomach . . . "
"In your chest?"
"Yes."
"Who did you see then?"
"Oh, I will find the letter the Dr. gave me."
"How is it now?"
"It's better, but I still feel something in my chest."
"Congested? Do you cough up phlegm? What color was it?"
[D asked where she was living.]
"River Park. I live on the top floor with friends from church living downstairs."
"Do you work?"
"Yes, as a nurse's aide in a nursing home. . . . It's not like it is back home. It's hard to work there; I'm working too hard." (p. 921)

At this point the authors noted that the patient demonstrated a shift in the intensity of her speech, a looking down to her left and a sinking-in-on-herself. Her saying "It's not like it is back home" conveyed a sense of complete despair. The comment was initially ignored by the resident, who next asked what if any additional symptoms the woman was experiencing. The patient reported pain and heavy bleeding associated with her periods and the interview ended. The patient's reference to home was charted as evidence of depression within a biomedical context and left at that.

The phrase "It's not like it is back home" has far different potential from a biopsychosocial standpoint. Now it is necessary to know what the phrase means to the patient. Does it mean that she would receive different treatment in Haiti? Could she receive the same type of help here? Questions need to be asked that facilitate a two-way exchange and also identify experiences the patient has had with her body, both positive and negative. This idea is demonstrated later in the interview:

D began by asking:
"You spoke of things being different back home . . . in terms of medicine . . . what do you do in Haiti?"
[. . . And in the course of the telling, B not just brightened but shifted her whole demeanor and stance; where just before she had appeared depressed and disconnected, now she became energized and present.]
B: " . . . Well maybe its not different in the city, in the hospital, they are all the same. But if you go out into the countryside, there are herbs

from the forest and Drs. who give massage and herbal wraps. My mother and family massage me. You have to go for three weeks. Here, not just anyone can touch you, they can pray with you, but not touch you."

"Why did you come to Boston?" asked D.

"My father brought me to NY and then I moved to Boston because I was engaged and my boyfriend's family lives in Boston. But we broke up 2 years ago."

"That's hard," said D, "and also not to have your family close by."

"Yes, that's when my problem began. And that's when I went to the doctor."

In this way she was slowly able to tell her story and to relate her medical problems to her sense of herself as a person and her personal world. (pp. 923–924)

The resident who witnessed this transformation through interviewing remarked: "You know, you get so entrenched in the biomedical, not wanting to keep any patient waiting, that you lose sight of the person." In this example a routine medical examination was transformed into a relational event in which the patient came to feel involved and respected rather than objectified and pathologized. The physician was also able to identify some nondrug therapies such as massage that the patient might be encouraged to seek out in her new culture.

Through the use of ordinary language and questions, the physician was able to create a collaborative healing environment between himself and his patient. Through this type of questioning, patients are invited as persons into equal partnership with their health care providers. Although this woman was expressing loneliness and a longing for a previous way of life, her chest and gynecological symptoms required treatment. She needed a perspective for understanding how to manage herself in the here and now. It would have been unfortunate if she had been simply diagnosed as depressed, given an antidepressant, and sent home. From a somatic awareness perspective, she needed to connect her feelings of loneliness and sadness to her bodily sensations and then learn to find ways to manage both. The question as to how she would have been treated in Haiti represented an insightful initial probe for developing a somatic awareness discourse with this patient. Her mood and outlook "brightened" following the question, and her response provided some important insight with respect to how best to initiate somatic awareness with her. She described massage and herbal wraps as basic to her healing heritage. The use of actual and/or symbolic variants of these forms of self-soothing represent an excellent starting point for initiating a course of treatment based on somatic awareness. This approach is not insensitive to the fact that her symptoms began with the loss of a relationship. The fact is that she must move on; the longer the bodily symptoms remain unmanaged, the greater the likelihood that they might become chronic in function.

The concept of somatic awareness represents a holistic and flexible heuristic for harnessing the healing capacity of the mind and body. The concept is applicable to a wide variety of chronic symptom and illness conditions and is compatible with most conventional and nonconventional treatments. Somatic awareness serves to directly involve patients in the understanding and management of their condition. The individual with migraine or other psychophysiological disorders can recognize and utilize bodily events that reduce susceptibility to a symptom episode. Even if unable to prevent a particular episode, they have the means, through the longer term development of somatic awareness, to make changes within themselves to reduce the likelihood of future symptom episodes. The need for bodily monitoring and regulation is equally true for individuals with serious illnesses, including arthritis, multiple sclerosis, and cancer. Utilizing somatic awareness in the face of progressive and/or life-threatening disease represents a considerable challenge, requiring the use of all the inner and external resources the individual can harness. We saw, however, that many individuals have discovered ways within themselves to stabilize and even reverse disease processes. These individuals represent living proof that the further study and application of somatic awareness in health care is greatly needed. Somatic awareness and the accompanying psychobiological perspective are well suited for directing future developments in holistic health.

References

Afable, R. F., & Ettinger, R. H. (1993). Musculoskeletal disease in the aged: Diagnosis and management. *Drugs and Aging, 3,* 49–59.

Alexander, F. (1950). *Psychosomatic medicine: Its principles and applications.* New York: Norton.

American College of Rheumatology Ad Hoc Committee on Clinical Guidelines. (1996). Guidelines for the management of rheumatoid arthritis. *Arthritis and Rheumatism, 39,* 713–722.

American Psychiatric Association. (1994). *Diagnostic and statistical manual of mental disorders* (4th ed.). Washington, DC: Author.

Amery, W. K., Waelkens, J., & Vandenbergh, V. (1986). Migraine warnings. *Headache, 26,* 60–66.

Antonovsky, A. (1994). A sociological critique of the "well-being" movement. *Advances, 10,* 6–12.

Asmundson, G. J. G., Norton, G. R., Wilson, K. G., & Sandler, L. S. (1994). Subjective symptoms and cardiac reactivity to brief hyperventilation in individuals with high anxiety sensitivity. *Behaviour Research and Therapy, 32,* 237–241.

Bain, A. (1855). *The senses and the intellect.* London: Parker & Son.

Bakal, D. (1982). *The psychobiology of chronic headache.* New York: Springer.

Bakal, D. (1992). *Psychology and health* (2nd ed.). New York: Springer.

Bakal, D., Demjen, S., & Duckro, P. (1994). Chronic daily headache and the elusive nature of somatic awareness. In R. C. Grzesiak & D. S. Ciccone (Eds.), *Psychological vulnerability to chronic pain* (pp. 116–136). New York: Springer.

Bakal, D., Fung, T., & Hesson, K. (1996). Heart rate, breathing, and subjective responses of a limited-symptom panic patient to 35% carbon dioxide challenge. *Canadian Journal of Psychiatry, 41,* 669–670.

Banks, S. M., & Kerns, R. D. (1996). Explaining high rates of depression in chronic pain: A diathesis-stress framework. *Psychological Bulletin, 119*, 95–110.

Baron, R. S., Cutrona, C. E., Hicklin, D., Russell, D. W., & Lubaroff, D. M. (1990). Social support and immune function among spouses of cancer patients. *Journal of Personality and Social Psychology, 59*, 344–352.

Barsky, A. J. (1992). Palpitations, cardiac awareness, and panic disorder. *American Journal of Medicine, 92*(Suppl. 1A), 31–35.

Basbaum, A. I. (1995). Insights into the development of opioid tolerance. *Pain, 61*, 349–352.

Bass, C. (1992). Chest pain and breathlessness: Relationship to psychiatric illness. *American Journal of Medicine, 92*(Suppl. 1A), 12–17.

Baumann, L. J., & Leventhal, H. (1985). "I can tell when my blood pressure is up, can't I?" *Health Psychology, 4*, 203–218.

Beck, A. T., & Emery, G. (1985). *Anxiety disorders and phobias: A cognitive perspective.* New York: Basic Books.

Beck, A. T., & Steer, R. A. (1990). *Manual for the Beck Anxiety Inventory.* San Antonio, TX: Psychological Corporation.

Beck, A. T., Steer, R. A., & Beck, J. S. (1993). Types of self-reported anxiety in outpatients with DSM-III-R anxiety disorders. *Anxiety, Stress, and Coping, 6*, 43–55.

Beecher, H. K. (1955). The powerful placebo. *Journal of the American Medical Association, 159*, 1602–1606.

Beecher, H. K. (1959). *Measurement of subjective responses: Quantitative effects of drugs.* New York: Oxford University Press.

Bennett, R. M. (1996). Fibromyalgia and the disability dilemma. *Arthritis and Rheumatism, 39*, 1627–1634.

Benson, H. (1996). *Timeless healing: The power and biology of belief.* New York: Scribners.

Benson, H., Beary, J. E., & Carol, M. P. (1974). The relaxation response. *Psychiatry, 37*, 37–46.

Berland, W. (1995). Unexpected cancer recovery: Why patients believe they survive. *Advances, 11*, 5–19.

Blau, J. N. (1990). Migraine theory and therapy: Their relationship. *Headache Quarterly: Current Treatment and Research, 1*, 15–22.

Block, K. I. (1997). The role of self in healthy cancer survivorship: A view from the front lines of treating cancer. *Advances, 13*, 6–26.

Boadella, D. (1994). Styles of breathing in Reichian therapy. In B. H. Timmons & R. Ley (Eds.), *Behavioral and psychological approaches to breathing disorders* (pp. 233–242). New York: Plenum Press.

Bolletino, R., & LeShan, L. (1995). Cancer patients and "marathon" psychotherapy: A new model. *Advances, 11*, 19–20.

Boring, E. G. (1942). *Sensation and perception in the history of experimental psychology.* New York: Appleton-Century-Crofts.

Boyd, J. H., & Crump, T. (1991). Westphal's agoraphobia. *Journal of Anxiety Disorders, 5*, 77–86.

Brehm, N. M., & Khantzian, E. J. (1992). A psychodynamic perspective. In J. H. Lowinson, P. Ruiz, & R. B. Millman (Eds.), *Substance abuse: A comprehensive textbook* (2nd ed., pp. 106–117). Baltimore: Williams & Wilkins.

Brown, B. B. (1980). *Supermind: The ultimate energy.* New York: Harper & Row.

Buchholz, I. (1994). Breathing, voice, and movement therapy: Applications to breathing disorders. *Biofeedback and Self-Regulation, 19,* 141–153.

Buchholz, W. M. (1997). The role of the physician in healthy cancer survivorship. *Advances, 13,* 30–33.

Burckhardt, C. S., Clark, S. R., O'Reilly, C. A., & Bennett, R. M. (1997). Pain-coping strategies of women with fibromyalgia: Relationship to pain, fatigue, and quality of life. *Journal of Musculoskeletal Pain, 5,* 5–21.

Callahan, L. F. (1996). Editorial: Arthritis as a women's health issue. *Arthritis Care and Research, 9,* 159–162.

Cantwell-Simmons, E., Duckro, P. N., & Richardson, W. D. (1993). A review of studies on the relationship of chronic analgesic use and chronic headaches. *Headache Quarterly, 4,* 28–35.

Cassell, E. J. (1976). Disease as an "it": Concepts of disease revealed by patients' presentations of symptoms. *Social Science and Medicine, 10,* 143–146.

Cassidy, C. M. (1994). Unraveling the ball of string: Reality, paradigms, and the study of alternative medicine. *Advances, 10,* 5–31.

Challis, G. B., & Stam, H. J. (1990). The spontaneous regression of cancer. *Acta Oncologica, 29,* 545–550.

Chambless, D. L., Caputo, G. C., Jasin, S. E., Gracely, E. J., & Williams, C. (1985). The Mobility Inventory for Agoraphobia. *Behaviour Research and Therapy, 23,* 35–44.

Chandra, F. A. (1994). Respiratory practices in yoga. In B. H. Timmons & R. Ley (Eds.), *Behavioral and psychological approaches to breathing disorders* (pp. 221–232). New York: Plenum Press.

Childress, A. R., Ehrman, R., Rohsenow, D. J., Robbins, S. J., & O'Brien, C. P. (1992). Classically conditioned factors in drug dependence. In J. H. Lowinson, P. Ruiz, & R. B. Millman (Eds.), *Substance abuse: A comprehensive textbook* (2nd ed., pp. 56–69). Baltimore: Williams & Wilkins.

Cioffi, D. (1991). Beyond attentional strategies: A cognitive-perceptual model of somatic interpretation. *Psychological Bulletin, 109,* 25–41.

Cohen, S., & Herbert, T. B. (1996). Health psychology: Psychological factors and physical disease from the perspective of human psychoneuroimmunology. *Annual Review of Psychology, 47,* 113–142.

Cole, S. W., Kemeny, M. E., & Taylor, S. E. (1997). Social identity and physical health: Accelerated HIV progression in rejection-sensitive gay men. *Journal of Personality and Social Psychology, 72,* 320–335.

Costa, P. T. Jr., & McCrae, R. R. (1987). Neuroticism, somatic complaints, and disease: Is the bark worse than the bite? *Journal of Personality, 55,* 299–316.

Cox, B. J., Cohen, E., Direnfeld, D. M., & Swinson, R. P. (1996). Does the Beck Anxiety Inventory measure anything beyond panic attack symptoms? *Behaviour Research and Therapy, 34,* 949–954.

Dafter, R. E. (1996). Shifts of core emotional self-experience: Can they influence cancer outcomes? *Advances, 12,* 62–71.

Devins, G. M., Edworthy, S. M., Guthrie, N. G., & Martin, L. (1992). Illness intrusiveness in rheumatoid arthritis: Differential impact on depressive symptoms over the adult lifespan. *Journal of Rheumatology, 19,* 709–715.

Diamond, E. L., Massey, K. L., & Covey, D. (1989). Symptom awareness and blood glucose estimation in diabetic adults. *Health Psychology, 8,* 15–26.

Diener, H. C., Dichgans, J., Scholz, E., Geiselhart, S., Gerber, W. D., & Bille, A. (1989). Analgesic-induced chronic headache: Long-term results of withdrawal therapy. *Journal of Neurology, 236,* 9–14.

Dienstfrey, H. (1997). Editorial. *Advances, 13,* 5.

Donovan, D. M. (1988). Assessment of addictive behaviors: Implications of an emerging biopsychosocial model. In D. M. Donovan & G. A. Marlatt (Eds.), *Assessment of addictive behaviors* (pp. 2–48). New York: Guilford Press.

Drachman, D. A., & Hart, C. W. (1972). An approach to the dizzy patient. *Neurology, 22,* 323–334.

Dracup, K., Moser, D. K., Eisenberg, M., Meischke, H., Alonzo, A. A., & Braslow, A. (1995). Causes of delay in seeking treatment for heart attack symptoms. *Social Science and Medicine, 40,* 379–392.

Droste, C., Greenlee, M. W., & Roskamm, H. (1986). A defective angina pectoris pain warning system: Experimental findings of ischemic and electrical pain test. *Pain, 26,* 199–209.

Duval, S., & Wicklund, R. A. (1972). *A theory of objective self-awareness.* New York: Academic Press.

Egger, L., Bakal, D., Fung, T. (1998). [Factor structure of the Beck Anxiety Inventory based on a student population.] Unpublished raw data.

Engel, G. L. (1959). "Psychogenic" pain and the pain-prone patient. *American Journal of Medicine, 26,* 899–918.

Engel, G. L. (1997). From biomedical to biopsychosocial: 1. Being scientific in the human domain. *Psychotherapy and Psychosomatics, 66,* 57–62.

Epstein, A. H. (1989). *Mind, fantasy, and healing: One woman's journey from conflict and illness to wholeness and health.* New York: Delacorte Press.

Evans, F. J. (1974). The placebo response in pain reduction. *Advances in Neurology, 4,* 289–296.

Evers, K. J., & Karnilowicz, W. (1996). Patient attitude as a function of disease state in multiple sclerosis. *Social Science and Medicine, 43,* 1245–1251.

Fawzy, F. I., Cousins, N., Fawzy, N. W., Kemeny, M. E., Elashoff, R., & Morton, D. (1990a). A structured psychiatric intervention for cancer patients: I. Changes over time in methods of coping and affective disturbance. *Archives of General Psychiatry, 47,* 720–725.

Fawzy, F. I., Kemeny, M. E., Fawzy, N. W., Elashoff, R., Morton, D., Cousins, N., & Fahey, J. L. (1990b). A structured psychiatric intervention for cancer patients: II. Changes over time in immunological measures. *Archives of General Psychiatry, 47,* 729–735.

Feldenkrais, M. (1972). *Awareness through movement.* New York: Harper & Row.

Fewtrell, W. D., & O'Connor, K. P. (1988). Dizziness and depersonalization. *Advances in Behavior Research and Therapy, 10,* 201–218,

Fine, P. G., Roberts, W. J., Gillette, R. G., & Child, T. R. (1994). Slowly developing placebo responses confound tests of intravenous phentolamine to determine mechanisms underlying idiographic chronic low back pain. *Pain, 56,* 235–242.

Fisher, S. (1986). *Development and structure of the body image* (Vol. 1). Hillsdale, NJ: Erlbaum.

Fisher, S., & Greenberg, R. P. (1989). A second opinion: Rethinking the claims of biological psychiatry. In S. Fisher & R. P. Greenberg (Eds.), *The limits of biological treatments for psychological distress* (pp. 309–336). Hillsdale, NJ: Erlbaum.

Fisk, J. D., Pontefract, A., Ritvo, P. G., Archibald, C. J., & Murray, T. J. (1994). The impact of fatigue on patients with multiple sclerosis. *Canadian Journal of Neurological Sciences, 24,* 9–14.

Fordyce, W. E. (1995). What is pain? In W. E. Fordyce (Ed.), *Back pain in the workplace* (pp. 11–17). Seattle: IASP Press.

Foss, L. (1996). Advancing psychosocial health education: A review of the Pew–Fetzer Report. *Advances, 12,* 43–50.

Frasure-Smith, N. (1987). Levels of somatic awareness in relation to angiographic findings. *Journal of Psychosomatic Research, 31,* 545–554.

Freedland, K. E., Carney, R. M., Krone, R. J., Smith, L. J., Rich, M. W., Eisenkramer, G., & Fischer, K. C. (1991). Psychological factors in silent myocardial ischemia. *Psychosomatic Medicine, 53,* 13–24.

Fried, R. (1993). *The psychology and physiology of breathing.* New York: Plenum Press.

Fritz, G. F., Rubinstein, S., & Lewiston, N. J. (1987). Psychological factors in fatal childhood asthma. *American Journal of Orthopsychiatry, 57,* 253–257.

Gallego, J., & Perruchet, P. (1991). Effect of practice on the voluntary control of a learned breathing pattern. *Physiology and Behavior, 49,* 315–319.

Gibbons, F. X. (1991). Self-evaluation and self-perception: The role of attention in the experience of anxiety. In R. Schwarzer & R. A. Wicklund (Eds.), *Anxiety and self-focused attention* (pp. 15–25). New York: Harwood Academic.

Glass, R. M. (1996). The patient–physician relationship: JAMA focuses on the center of medicine. *Journal of the American Medical Association, 275,* 147–148.

Goldberger, A. L. (1996). Comments on energy cardiology: A dynamical systems approach for integrating conventional and alternative medicine. *Advances, 12,* 31–32.

Goldstein, A. J., & Chambless, D. L. (1978). A reanalysis of agoraphobia. *Behavior Therapy, 9,* 47–59.

Gordon, E. E. (1996). The placebo: An insight into mind–body interaction. *Headache Quarterly: Current Treatment and Research, 7,* 117–125.

Grant, I., Brown, G. W., Harris, T., McDonald, W. I., Patterson, T., & Trimble, M. R. (1989). Severely threatening events and marked life difficulties preceding onset or exacerbation of multiple sclerosis. *Journal of Neurology, Neurosurgery, and Psychiatry, 52,* 8–13.

Greenberg, R. P., Bornstein, R. F., Zborowski, M. J., Fisher, S., & Greenberg, M. D. (1994). A meta-analysis of fluoxetine outcome in the treatment of depression. *Journal of Nervous and Mental Disease, 182,* 547–551.

Greenberg, R. P., & Fisher, S. (1989). Examining antidepressant effectiveness: Findings, ambiguities, and some vexing puzzles. In S. Fisher & R. P. Greenberg (Eds.), *The limits of biological treatments for psychological distress* (pp. 1–37). Hillsdale, NJ: Erlbaum.

Grünbaum, A. (1993). *Validation in the clinical theory of psychoanalysis.* Madison, CT: International Universities Press.

Hall, G., Compston, A., & Scolding, N. (1997). Beta-interferon and multiple sclerosis. *Trends in Neurosciences, 20,* 63–67.

Hanna, T. (1970, Autumn). The field of somatics. *Somatics,* pp. 30–34.

Hanna, T. (1988). *Somatics.* Reading, MA: Addison-Wesley.

Hannan, M. T. (1996). Epidemiologic perspectives on women and arthritis: An overview. *Arthritis Care and Research, 9,* 424–434.

Hansell, S., & Mechanic, D. (1991). Body awareness and self-assessed health among older adults. *Journal of Aging and Health, 3,* 473–492.

Heide, F. J., & Borkovec, T. D. (1984). Relaxation-induced anxiety: Mechanisms and theoretical explanations. *Behaviour Research and Therapy, 22,* 1–12

Heim, E., Blaser, A., & Waidelich, E. (1972). Dyspnea: Psychophysiologic relationships. *Psychosomatic Medicine, 34,* 405–423.

Hesson, K., Hill, T., & Bakal, D. (1997). Variability in breathing patterns during latent labor: A pilot study. *Journal of Nurse-Midwifery, 42,* 99–103.

Hilgard, E. R., & Hilgard, J. R. (1975). *Hypnosis in the relief of pain.* Los Altos, CA: Kaufman.

Horton, P. C. (1981). *Solace.* Chicago: University of Chicago Press.

Horton, P. C. (1988). Introduction. In P. C. Horton, H. Gewirtz, & K. J. Kreutter (Eds.), *The solace paradigm: An eclectic search for psychological immunity* (pp. 3–39). Madison, WI: International Universities Press.

House, J. S., Landis, K. R., & Umberson, D. (1988). Social relationships and health. *Science, 241,* 540–545.

Ikemi, Y., Nakagawa, S., Nakagawa, T., & Sugita, M. (1975). Psychosomatic consideration on cancer patients who have made a narrow escape from death. *Dynamische Psychiatrie, 8,* 77–92.

International Association for the Study of Pain. (1986). Classification of chronic pain: Description of chronic pain syndromes and definitions of pain terms, *Pain*(Suppl. 3), S1–S225.

Jaffe, J. H. (1992). Opiates: Clinical aspects. In J. H. Lowinson, P. Ruiz, & R. B. Millman (Eds.), *Substance abuse: A comprehensive textbook* (2nd ed., pp. 186–194). Baltimore: Williams & Wilkins.

Janca, A., Isaac, M., Bennett, L. A., & Tacchini, G. (1995). Somatoform disorders in different cultures: A mail questionnaire survey. *Social Psychiatry and Psychiatric Epidemiology, 30,* 44–48.

Jiang, W., Babyak, M., Krantz, D. S., Waugh, R. A., Coleman, R. E., Hanson, M. M., Frid, D. J., McNulty, S., Morris, J. J., O'Connor, C. M., & Blumenthal,

J. A. (1996). Mental stress-induced myocardial ischemia and cardiac events. *Journal of the American Medical Association, 275,* 1651–1656.

Joyce, J., Hotopf, M., & Wessely, S. (1997). The prognosis of chronic fatigue and chronic fatigue syndrome: A systematic review. *Quarterly Journal of Medicine, 90,* 223–233.

Julian, D. G. (1996). If I woke with central chest pain. . . . *Lancet, 348,* S29–S31.

Julien, R. M. (1995). *A primer of drug action* (7th ed.). New York: Freeman.

Kagan, J. (1994). *Galen's prophecy: Temperament in human nature.* New York: Basic Books.

Kaplan, G. (1995). Where do shared pathways lead? Some reflections on a research agenda. *Psychosomatic Medicine, 57,* 208–212.

Katz, A. M., & Shotter, J. (1996). Hearing the patient's "voice": Toward a social poetics in diagnostic interviews. *Social Science and Medicine, 43,* 919–931.

Kauhanen, J., Kaplan, G. A., Cohen, R. D., Julkunen, J., & Salonen, J. T. (1996). Alexithymia and risk of death in middle-aged men. *Journal of Psychosomatic Research, 41,* 541–549.

Keefe, F. J., Caldwell, D. S., Martinez, S., Nunley, J., Beckham, J., & Williams, D. A. (1991). Analyzing pain in rheumatoid arthritis patients: Pain coping strategies in patients who have had knee replacement surgery. *Pain, 46,* 153–160.

Kemeny, M. E. (1994). Psychoneuroimmunology of HIV infection. *Psychiatric Clinics of North America, 17,* 55–68.

Kemeny, M. E., Weiner, H., Duran, R., Taylor, S. E., Visscher, B., & Fahey, J. L. (1995). Immune system changes after the death of a partner in HIV-positive gay men. *Psychosomatic Medicine, 57,* 547–554.

Kennedy, B. L., & Schwab, J. J. (1997). Utilization of medical specialists by anxiety disorder patients. *Psychosomatics, 38,* 109–112.

Kiecolt-Glaser, J., & Glaser, R. (1988). Psychological influences on immunity. *American Psychologist, 43,* 892–898.

Kirmayer, L. J. (1984). Culture, affect, and somatization (Part I). *Transcultural Psychiatric Research Review, 21,* 159–188.

Kirschbaum, C., Klauer, T., Filipp, S. H., & Hellhammer, D. H. (1995). Sex-specific effects of social support on cortisol and subjective responses to acute psychological stress. *Psychosomatic Medicine, 57,* 23–31.

Klein, D. F. (1993). False suffocation alarms, spontaneous panics, and related conditions: An integrative hypothesis. *Archives of General Psychiatry, 50,* 306–317.

Krieger, N., & Sidney, S. (1996). Racial discrimination and blood pressure: The CARDIA study of young black and white adults. *American Journal of Public Health, 86,* 1370–1378.

Kroenke, K. (1992). Symptoms in medical patients: An untended field. *American Journal of Medicine, 92*(Suppl. 1A), 1–7.

Kroenke, K., & Mangelsdorff, A. D. (1989). Common symptoms in ambulatory care: Incidence, evaluation, therapy, and outcome. *American Journal of Medicine, 86,* 262–266.

Krystal, H. (1982). Alexithymia and the effectiveness of psychoanalytic treatment. *International Journal of Psychoanalytic Psychotherapy, 9,* 353–388.

Kushner, M. G., & Beitman, B. D. (1990). Panic attacks without fear: An overview. *Behaviour Research and Therapy, 28,* 469–479.

Kushner, M. G., Beitman, B. D., & Beck, N. C. (1989). Factors predictive of panic disorder in cardiology patients with chest pain and no evidence of coronary artery disease: A cross-validation. *Journal of Psychosomatic Research, 33,* 207–215.

Lechin, F., van der Dijs, B., & Benaim, M. (1996). Benzodiazepines: Tolerability in elderly patients. *Psychotherapy and Psychosomatics, 65,* 171–182.

Lehrer, P. M., Carr, R., Sargunaraj, D., & Woolfolk, R. L. (1994). Stress management techniques: Are they all equivalent, or do they have specific effects? *Biofeedback and Self-Regulation, 19,* 353–401.

Lerner, M. (1994). *Choices in healing.* Cambridge, MA: MIT Press.

Leserman, J., Drossman, D. A., Li, Z., Toomey, T. C., Nachman, G., & Glogau, L. (1996). Sexual and physical abuse history in gastroenterology practice: How types of abuse impact health status. *Psychosomatic Medicine, 58,* 4–15.

Leventhal, E. A., Leventhal, H., Shacham, S., & Easterling, D. V. (1989). Active coping reduces reports of pain from childbirth. *Journal of Consulting and Clinical Psychology, 57,* 365–371.

Leventhal, H. (1993). The pain system: A multilevel model for the study of motivation and emotion. *Motivation and Emotion, 17,* 139–146.

Levine, D. M., Green, L. W., Deeds, S. G., Chwalow, J., Russell, R. P., & Finlay, J. (1979). Health education for hypertensive patients. *Journal of the American Medical Association, 241,* 1700–1703.

Linton, S. J. (1997). A population-based study of the relationship between sexual abuse and back pain: Establishing a link. *Pain, 73,* 47–53.

Linzer, M., Pontinen, M., Gold, D. T., Divine, G. W., Felder, A., & Brooks, W. B. (1991). Impairment of physical and psychosocial function in recurrent syncope. *Journal of Clinical Epidemiology, 44,* 1037–1043.

Lloyd, R. (1996). New directions in psychoneuroimmunology: A critique. *Advances, 12,* 5–11.

Lorig, K., & Fries, J. F. (1995). *The arthritis helpbook: A tested self-management program for coping with arthritis and fibromyalgia.* Reading, MA: Addison-Wesley.

Lorig, K., Seleznick, M., Lubeck, D., Ung, E., Chastain, R. L., & Holman, H. R. (1989). The beneficial outcomes of the arthritis self-management course are not adequately explained by behavior change. *Arthritis and Rheumatism, 32,* 91–95.

Lowen, A. (1958). *The language of the body.* New York: Grune & Stratton.

Lumley, M. A., Stettner, L., & Wehmer, F. (1996). How are alexithymia and physical illness linked? A review and critique of pathways. *Journal of Psychosomatic Research, 41,* 505–518.

Lundh, L. (1987). Placebo, belief, and health. A cognitive-emotional model. *Scandinavian Journal of Psychology, 28,* 128–143.

Lyman, B., & Waters, J. C. E. (1986). The experiential loci and sensory qualities of various emotions. *Motivation and Emotion, 10,* 25–37.

Lynch, P., Bakal, D. A., Whitelaw, W., & Fung, T. (1991). Chest muscle activity and panic anxiety: A preliminary investigation. *Psychosomatic Medicine, 53,* 80–89.

Maier, S. F., Watkins, L. R., & Fleshner, M. (1994). Psychoneuroimmunology: The interface between behavior, brain, and immunity. *American Psychologist, 49,* 1004–1017.

Mandler, G., Mandler, J. M., & Uviller, E. T. (1958). Autonomic feedback: The perception of autonomic activity. *Journal of Abnormal and Social Psychology, 56,* 367–373.

Mao, J., Price, D. D., & Mayer, D. J. (1995). Experimental mononeuropathy reduces the antinociceptive effects of morphine: Implications for common intracellular mechanisms involved in morphine tolerance and neuropathic pain. *Pain, 61,* 353–364.

Matsumi, J. T., & Draguns, J. G. (1996). Culture and psychopathology. In J. W. Berry, M. H. Segall, & C. Kagitcibasi (Eds.), *Handbook of cross-cultural psychology* (2nd ed.): *Vol. 3. Social behavior and applications* (pp. 449–491). Needham Heights, MA: Allyn & Bacon.

Matthews, D. A., Suchman, A. L., & Branch, W. T. (1993). Making "connexions": Enhancing the therapeutic potential of patient–clinician relationships. *Annals of Internal Medicine, 118,* 973–977.

McCraty, R., Atkinson, M., Tiller, W. A., Rein, G., & Watkins, A. D. (1995). The effects of emotions on short-term power spectrum analysis of heart rate variability. *American Journal of Cardiology, 76,* 1089–1092.

McDonald, W. I., Miller, D. H., & Thompson, A. J. (1994). Are magnetic resonance findings predictive of clinical outcome in therapeutic trials in multiple sclerosis?: The dilemma of Interferon-B. *Annals of Neurology, 36,* 14–18.

McEwan, B. S., & Stellar, E. (1993). Stress and the individual. *Archives of Internal Medicine, 153,* 2093–2101.

McLaughlin, J., & Zeeberg, I. (1993). Self-care and multiple sclerosis: A view from two cultures. *Social Science and Medicine, 37,* 315–329.

McMahon, S. B., Lewin, G. R., & Wall, P. D. (1993). Central hyperexcitability triggered by noxious inputs. *Current Opinion in Neurobiology, 3,* 602–610.

Melzack, R. (1984). The myth of painless childbirth [The John J. Bonica Lecture]. *Pain, 19,* 321–337.

Melzack, R. (1990a). Phantom limbs and the concept of a neuromatrix. *Trends in Neurosciences, 13,* 88–92.

Melzack, R. (1990b). The tragedy of needless pain. *Scientific American, 262,* 27–33.

Merskey, H. (1996). Plenary session on fibromyalgia: Introduction. *Pain Research and Management, 1,* 41.

Merskey, H., & Bogduk, N. (1994). *Classification of chronic pain: Description of chronic pain syndromes and definitions of pain terms* (2nd ed.). Seattle: IASP Press.

Miller, L. C., Murphy, R., & Buss, A. H. (1981). Consciousness of body: Private and public. *Journal of Personality and Social Psychology, 41,* 397–406.

Miller-Blair, D. J., & Robbins, D. L. (1993). Rheumatoid arthritis: New science, new treatment. *Geriatrics, 48,* 28–38.

Moldofsky, H. (1989). Nonrestorative sleep and symptoms after a febrile illness in patients with fibrositis and chronic fatigue syndrome. *Journal of Rheumatology, 19*(Suppl.), 150–153.

Morgan, W., & Pollock, M. (1977). Psychologic characterization of the elite distance runner. *Annals of the New York Academy of Sciences, 301,* 382–403.

Motz, J. (1996). What energy "knows." *Advances, 12,* 33.

Naifeh, K. H. (1994). Basic anatomy and physiology of the respiratory system and the autonomic nervous system. In B. H. Timmons & R. Ley (Eds.), *Behavioral and psychological approaches to breathing disorders* (pp. 17–45). New York: Plenum Press.

Nemiah, J. C. (1996). Alexithymia: Present, past–future? *Psychosomatic Medicine, 58,* 217–218.

O'Regan, B., & Hirshberg, C. (1993). *Spontaneous remission: An annotated bibliography.* Bolinas, CA: Institute of Noetic Sciences.

Ornstein, R., & Sobel, D. (1987). *The healing brain.* New York: Simon & Schuster.

Ots, T. (1990). The angry liver, the anxious heart, and the melancholy spleen. *Culture, Medicine, and Psychiatry, 14,* 21–58.

Ottaviani, R., & Beck, A. T. (1987). Cognitive aspects of panic disorders. *Journal of Anxiety Disorders, 1,* 15–28.

Otto, H. A. (1966). *Explorations in human potentialities.* Springfield, IL: Charles C Thomas.

Otto, M. W., Pollack, M. H., Meltzer-Brody, S., & Rosenbaum, J. F. (1992). Cognitive-behavioral therapy for benzodiazepine discontinuation in panic disorder patients. *Psychopharmacology Bulletin, 28,* 123–130.

Patel, C. (1994). Foreword. In B. H. Timmons & R. Ley (Eds.), *Behavioral and psychological approaches to breathing disorders* (pp. ix–x). New York: Plenum Press.

Pawlikowska, T., Chalder, T., Hirsch, S. R., Wallace, P., Wright, D. J. M., & Wessely, S. C. (1994). Population-based study of fatigue and psychological distress. *British Medical Journal, 308,* 763–766.

Pennebaker, J. W., & Watson, D. (1988). Blood pressure estimation and beliefs among normotensives and hypertensives. *Health Psychology, 7,* 309–328.

Pennisi, E. (1997). Tracing molecules that make the brain–body connection. *Science, 275,* 930–931.

Pesso, A. (1969). *Movement in psychotherapy.* New York: New York University Press.

Piccinelli, M., & Simon, G. (1997). Gender and cross-cultural differences in somatic symptoms associated with emotional distress: An international study in primary care. *Psychological Medicine, 27,* 433–444.

Pincus, T. (1996). Book review of *Spontaneous remission: An annotated biography. Advances, 12,* 64–69.

Plotkin, W. B. (1985). A psychological approach to placebo: The role of faith in therapy and treatment. In L. White, B. Tursky, & G. E. Schwartz (Eds.), *Placebo: Theory, research, and mechanisms* (pp. 237–254). New York: Guilford Press.

Portenoy, R. K. (1996). Opioid therapy for chronic nonmalignant pain. *Pain Research and Management, 1,* 17–28.

Portenoy, R. K., & Payne, R. (1992). Acute and chronic pain. In J. H. Lowinson,

P. Ruiz, & R. B. Millman (Eds.), *Substance abuse: A comprehensive textbook* (2nd ed., pp. 691–721). Baltimore: Williams & Wilkins.

Poser, C. M. (1994). Multiple sclerosis: Diagnosis and treatment. *Medical Principles and Practice, 3,* 1–16.

Prochaska, J. O. (1995). Why do people behave the way we do? *Canadian Journal of Cardiology, 11*(Suppl. A), 20–25.

Pyszczynski, T., Greenberg, J., Solomon, S., & Hamilton, J. (1991). A terror management analysis of self-awareness and anxiety: The hierarchy of terror. In R. Schwarzer & R. A. Wicklund (Eds.), *Anxiety and self-focused attention* (pp. 67–85). New York: Harwood Academic.

Rabins, P. V., Brooks, B. R., O'Donell, P., Pearlson, G. D., Moberg, P., Jubelt, B., Coyle, P., Dalos, N., & Folstein, M. F. (1986). Structural brain correlates of emotional disorder in multiple sclerosis. *Brain, 109,* 585–597.

Reich, W. (1942). *The function of the orgasm.* New York: Orgone Institute Press.

Reich, W. (1962). *Character-analysis* (3rd ed.). New York: Noonday Press.

Ribot, T. (1884). The diseases of personality. In D. N. Robinson (Ed.). *Significant contributions to the history of psychology, 1750–1920* (pp. 1–163). Washington, DC: University Publications of America.

Roberts, A. H., Kewman, D. G., Mercier, L., & Hovell, M. (1993). The power of nonspecific effects in healing: Implications for psychosocial and biological treatments. *Clinical Psychology Review, 13,* 375–391.

Rosenbaum, J. F. (1987). Limited-symptom panic attacks. *Psychosomatics, 28,* 407–412.

Rosenthal, T. L. (1993). To soothe the savage breast. *Behaviour Research and Therapy, 31,* 439–462.

Rosomoff, H. L., Fishbain, D. A., Goldberg, M., Santana, R., & Rosomoff, R. S. (1989). Physical findings in patients with chronic intractable benign pain of the neck and/or back. *Pain, 37,* 279–287.

Russek, L. G., & Schwartz, G. E. (1996). Energy cardiology: A dynamical energy systems approach for integrating conventional and alternative medicine. *Advances, 12,* 4–24.

Russek, L. G., & Schwartz, G. E. (1997). Feelings of parental caring predict health status in midlife: A 35-year follow-up of the Harvard Mastery of Stress Study. *Journal of Behavioral Medicine, 20,* 1–13.

Salaffi, F., Cavalieri, F., Nolli, M., & Ferraccioli, G. (1991). Analysis of disability in knee osteoarthritis: Relationship with age and psychological variables but not with radiographic score. *Journal of Rheumatology, 18,* 1581–1585.

Sapirstein, G., & Kirsch, I. (1996, August). *Listening to Prozac, but hearing placebo?: A meta analysis of the placebo effect of antidepressant medication.* Paper presented at the 104th annual convention of the American Psychological Association, Toronto, Canada.

Schachter, S., & Singer, J. E. (1962). Cognitive, social, and physiological determinants of emotional state. *Psychological Review, 69,* 379–399.

Schwartz, M. S., & Associates. (1995). *Biofeedback: A practitioner's guide* (2nd ed.). New York: Guilford Press.

Seeman, T. E., & McEwan, B. S. (1996). Impact of social environment characteristics on neuroendocrine regulation. *Psychosomatic Medicine, 58,* 459–471.

Shapiro, A. K., & Morris, L. A. (1978). The placebo effect in medical and psychological therapies. In A. E. Bergin & S. L. Garfield (Eds.), *Handbook of psychotherapy and behavior change: An empirical analysis* (pp. 369–410). New York: Wiley.

Shields, S. A., Mallory, M. E., & Simon, A. (1989). The Body Awareness Questionnaire: Reliability and validity. *Journal of Personality Assessment, 53,* 802–815.

Shields, S. A., & Simon, A. (1991). Is awareness of bodily change in emotion related to awareness of other bodily processes? *Journal of Personality Assessment, 57,* 96–109.

Shug, S. A., & Large, R. G. (1995). Opioids for chronic noncancer pain. *Pain: Clinical Updates, 3,* 1–4.

Sifneos, P. E. (1973). The prevalence of "alexithymic" characteristics in psychosomatic patients. *Psychotherapy and Psychosomatics, 22,* 255–262.

Sifneos, P. E. (1996). Alexithymia: Past and present. *American Journal of Psychiatry, 153,* 137–142.

Simon, G. E. (1991). Somatization and psychiatric disorders. In L. J. Kirmayer & J. M. Robbins (Eds.), *Current concepts of somatization: Research and clinical perspectives* (pp. 37–62). Washington, DC: American Psychiatric Press.

Simon, G. E., & Von Korff, M. (1991). Somatization and psychiatric disorders in the NIMH Epidemiologic Catchment Area Study. *American Journal of Psychiatry, 148,* 1494–1500.

Skerritt, P. W. (1983). Anxiety and the heart: A historical review. *Psychological Medicine, 13,* 17–25.

Slater, E., & Roth, M. (1969). *Clinical psychiatry* (3rd ed.). London: Bailliere, Tindall, & Cassell.

Smith, C. A., & Wallston, K. A. (1992). Adaptation in patients with rheumatoid arthritis: Application of a general model. *Health Psychology, 11,* 151–162.

Sperry, R. W. (1987). Structure and significance of the consciousness revolution. *Journal of Mind and Behavior, 8,* 37–65.

Sperry, R. (1988). Psychology's mentalist paradigm and the religion/science tension. *American Psychologist, 43,* 607–613.

Spiegel, D., Bloom, J., Kraemer, H. C., & Gottheil, E. (1989). Effect of psychosocial treatment on survival of patients with metastatic breast cancer. *Lancet, 2,* 888–891.

Steptoe, A., & Noll, A. (1997). The perception of bodily sensations, with special reference to hypochondriasis. *Behaviour Research and Therapy, 35,* 910–910.

Steptoe, A., & Vögele, C. (1992). Individual differences in the perception of bodily sensations: The role of trait anxiety and coping style. *Behaviour Research and Therapy, 30,* 597–607.

Stewart, M. A. (1995). Effective physician–patient communication and health outcomes: A review. *Canadian Medical Association Journal, 152,* 1423–1433.

Sullivan, M. D. (1993). Placebo controls and epistemic control in orthodox medicine. *Journal of Medicine and Philosophy, 18*, 213–231.

Sulloway, F. J. (1979). *Freud, biologist of the mind.* New York: Basic Books.

Swinson, R. P., Cox, B. J., Shulman, I. D., Kuch, K., & Woszczyna, C. B. (1992). Medication use and the assessment of agoraphobic avoidance. *Behaviour Research and Therapy, 30*, 563–568.

Taylor, S. E., Repetti, R. L., & Seeman, T. (1997). Health psychology: What is an unhealthy environment and how does it get under the skin? *Annual Review of Psychology, 48*, 411–447.

Telch, M. J., Brouillard, M., Telch, C. F., Agras, W. S., & Taylor, C. B. (1989). Role of cognitive appraisal in panic-related avoidance. *Behaviour Research and Therapy, 27*, 373–383.

Temoshok, L. (1990). On attempting to articulate the biopsychosocial model: Psychological-psychophysiological homeostasis. In H. S. Friedman (Ed.), *Personality and disease* (pp. 203–225). New York: Wiley.

Theorell, T., Blomkvist, V., Jonsson, H., Schulman, S., Berntorp, E., & Stigendal, L. (1995). Social support and the development of immune function in human immunodeficiency virus infection. *Psychosomatic Medicine, 57*, 32–36.

Thomson, R. (1982). Side effects and placebo amplification. *British Journal of Psychiatry, 140*, 64–68.

Timmons, B. H. (1994). Breathing-related issues in therapy. In B. H. Timmons & R. Ley (Eds.), *Behavioral and psychological approaches to breathing disorders* (pp. 261–292). New York: Plenum Press.

Torosian, T., Lumley, M. A., Pickard, S. D., & Ketterer, M. W. (1997). Silent versus symptomatic myocardial ischemia: The role of psychological and medical factors. *Health Psychology, 16*, 123–130.

Tung, M. P. M. (1994). Symbolic meanings of the body in Chinese culture and "somatization." *Culture, Medicine, and Psychiatry, 18*, 483–492.

Tyrer, P., Murphy, S., & Riley, P. (1990). The Benzodiazepine Withdrawal Symptom Questionnaire. *Journal of Affective Disorders, 19*, 53–61.

Uchino, B. N., Cacioppo, J. T., & Kiecolt-Glaser, J. K. (1996). The relationship between social support and physiological processes: A review with emphasis on underlying mechanisms and implications for health. *Psychological Bulletin, 119*, 488–531.

Upledger, J. E. (1990). *SomatoEmotional release and beyond.* Palm Beach Gardens, FL: Upledger Institute.

Valins, S. (1967). Emotionality and information concerning internal reactions. *Journal of Personality and Social Psychology, 6*, 458–463.

van Baalen, D., de Vries, M., & Gondrie, M. (1987). *Psycho-social correlates of spontaneous regression in cancer* [Monograph]. Department of General Pathology, Medical Faculty, Erasmus University, Rotterdam, The Netherlands.

van der Feltz-Cornelis, C. M., & van Dyck, R. (1997). The notion of somatization: An artefact of the conceptualization of body and mind. *Psychotherapy and Psychosomatics, 66*, 117–127.

Vercoulen, J. H., Homes, O. R., Swanik, C. M., Jongen, P. J., Fennis, J. F.,

Galama, J. M., van der Meer, J. W., & Bleijenberg, G. (1996). The measurement of fatigue in patients with multiple sclerosis. *Archives of Neurology, 53,* 642–649.

Von Korff, M., Galer, B. S., & Stang, P. (1995). Chronic use of symptomatic headache medications. *Pain, 62,* 179–186.

Wall, P. D. (1992). The placebo effect: An unpopular topic. *Pain, 51,* 1–3.

Walls, E. W., & Philipp, E. E. (1953). *Hilton's rest and pain* (6th ed.). London: G. Bell & Sons. (Original work published 1863; London: Bell & Daldy)

Ware, N. C., & Kleinman, A. (1992). Culture and somatic experience: The social course of illness in neurasthenia and chronic fatigue syndrome. *Psychosomatic Medicine, 54,* 546–560.

Warren, S., Warren, K. G., & Cockerill, R. (1991). Emotional stress and coping in multiple sclerosis (MS) exacerbations. *Journal of Psychosomatic Research, 35,* 37–47.

Wegner, D. M., Broome, A., & Blumberg, S. J. (1997). Ironic effects of trying to relax under stress. *Behaviour Research and Therapy, 35,* 11–21.

Weiss, J. H. (1994). Behavioral management of asthma. In B. H. Timmons and R. Ley (Eds.), *Behavioral and psychological approaches to breathing disorders* (pp. 205–219). New York: Plenum Press.

Wickland, R. A. (1991). Introduction. In R. Schwarzer & R. A. Wicklund (Eds.), *Anxiety and self-focused attention* (pp. ix–xii). New York: Harwood Academic.

Wickramasekera, I. E. (1995). Somatization: Concepts, data, and predictions from the High Risk Model of Threat Perception. *Journal of Nervous and Mental Disease, 183,* 15–23.

Winnicott, D. W. (1953). Transitional objects and transitional phenomena. *International Journal of Psycho-Analysis, 34,* 89–97.

Wolfe, F., Hawley, D. J., & Wilson, K. (1996). The prevalence and meaning of fatigue in rheumatic disease. *Journal of Rheumatology, 23,* 1407–1417.

Wolff, H. G. (1937). Personality features and reactions of subjects with migraine. *Archives of Neurology, 37,* 895–921.

World Health Organization Expert Committee. (1990). *Cancer pain relief and palliative care.* Geneva: World Health Organization.

Wuitchik, M., Bakal, D., & Lipshitz, J. (1989). The clinical significance of pain and cognitive activity in latent labor. *Obstetrics and Gynecology, 73,* 35–42.

Yellowlees, P. M., & Kalucy, R. S. (1990). Psychobiological aspects of asthma and the consequent research implications. *Chest, 97,* 629–634.

Index